Natural Medicine

BRIAN INGLIS

FONTANA/COLLINS

First published by William Collins Sons
and Company Ltd 1979
First issued in Fontana Paperbacks 1980
Copyright © Brian Inglis 1979

Set in Linotype Times Roman

Made and printed in Great Britain by
William Collins Sons and Company Ltd, Glasgow

Contents

Introduction

When, twenty years ago, the late Geoffrey Murray undertook to survey unorthodox medical practices in Britain for the *Spectator* they were so little known that they had not acquired a collective name. With the Edinburgh Festival in mind he and I settled for 'Fringe Medicine', a term which was promptly adopted by the *British Medical Journal*.

While expressing scepticism about most of the therapies described, the *BMJ* editorial admitted 'we may have something to learn from the others'; and the intervening two decades have shown this to be an understatement. In some instances the change of status has been dramatic: notably in the case of acupuncture. So little notice had acupuncture attracted by 1959 that Murray did not even mention it. When, four years later, I wrote *Fringe Medicine* (he and I had been commissioned to produce the book together, but his job had taken him out of the country) I was advised even by people sympathetic to unorthodox therapies to leave acupuncture out, because it was so demonstrably bogus. But now . . .

Unorthodox forms of diagnosis and treatment today enjoy public confidence of a kind that then seemed hardly conceivable. Partly this is the consequence of growing dissatisfaction with orthodox medicine. Modern drugs, it has come to be realized, are not the answer to most of the diseases of civilisation – cancer, heart disorders, arthritis, allergies and the rest. The cost of orthodox treatment, too, has been mounting until in the United States it has become a source of alarm to the Federal Government, and to citizens compelled to set aside an ever-increasing proportion of their incomes for insurance. And although the cost has been kept under better control in Britain, the once admired National Health Service shows many signs of decay. 'Cash problems aside,' as an editorial in *World Medicine* observed on the occasion of the service's thirtieth anniversary, 'the NHS is drifting deeper into inertia, self-becalmed in part by its lost sense of direction.'

One prescription for such a lost sense of direction is a blood transfusion from the 'fringe'. The term, though, has had its day. The Italians, who have been the most vigorous campaigners on unorthodoxy's behalf, prefer 'the Other Medicine'. In France there has been a move to popularise 'Biotherapy'. The Americans call it 'Alternative Medicine', a version which has recently been establishing itself in Britain. The World Health Organisation has settled for 'Traditional Medicine'; and although it originally referred to indigenous practices in Africa, the definition – 'the sum total of all the knowledge and practices, whether explicable or not, used in diagnosis, prevention and elimination of physical, mental or social imbalance, and relying exclusively on practical experience and observation handed down from generation to generation, whether verbally or in writing' – until very recently applied to unorthodox theories and practices in Europe and America, too. But British practitioners now favour 'Natural Medicine' (or 'Natural Therapeutics'), designed to emphasise that they are the upholders of the Hippocratic view that nature has its own healing force, and that the aim of treatment should be to assist rather than to supplant it. And my aim has been to trace the devolopment of the theories and practices of natural medicine from their source in tribal communities up to the present.

'The present', though, gives rise to a problem. In *Fringe Medicine,* a journalist's eye view of the scene in the 1960s, it was easy to sort the alternative therapies out into a few well-defined categories. Today 'paramedical practitioners' – the term favoured by the British Department of Health – are increasingly being tempted to learn and practise a variety of methods. Old forms of therapy, too, are being imported, or revived, or adapted; and so rapid is the process of transformation that what is intended as a survey takes on the complexion of a running commentary.

It is partly for this reason that I have not attempted to assess the merits of the various therapies. In a period of such rapid expansion and cross-fertilisation this would hardly be feasible. But in any case it would be unwise. I have often been asked, particularly at medical gatherings, whether I 'believe in' osteopaths, or acupuncturists, or whatever group happens to be under discussion, and whether I myself go to them, rather than to a doctor. As it happens, I have no first-hand experience of any of them, except for purposes of demonstration; but even if I had, I would not feel justified in relying on it. My belief is that it is more sensible to seek whatever treatment may be required from individuals whose knowledge, skill and personality inspire confidence, whether they are medically qualified or not.

It is best, of course, not to have to seek treatment at all. There are many organisations which, though not primarily concerned with health, believe that the key to it can be found in their philosophy, or religion; but such teachings as An-throposophy, Sufism, Theosophy and Zen seemed to me to lie just outside of this book's scope. Some of them, though, have their own medical theories and practices. Information about them, and about other organisations in the field of natural medicine, is in the appendix.

Chapter One

EARLY MEDICINE

In ordinary conditions wild animals preserve their fitness instinctively, eating the kind of food which nourishes them, ignoring whatever is poisonous. Even sheep on farms, it has been found, can tell which segment of a pasture contains the trace elements necessary for their health; they will crop it first, before appeasing their hunger on the rest of the grass. But man has lost this ability, presumably as part of the price paid for becoming *homo sapiens*; for acquiring reasoning power. Tribal man began to rely on memory, rather than instinct, to tell him which berries were safe to eat, and from which springs it was safe to drink; decisions which were left to the elders of the tribe.

TRIBAL DOCTORS

There was, however, another health service available to him. If consciousness could be suspended for a while, instinct or intuition might provide the answers. An individual who could 'dissociate' – enter into a state of trance, in order to consult instinct – was consequently regarded as of great value to the tribe: the obvious choice, in fact, as tribal doctor. When explorers, missionaries, and traders began to describe what they had seen of tribal customs, their reports showed that tribes all over the world employed what they variously described as shamans, witch doctors or medicine men, chosen because of this ability.

Sometimes the tribal doctor would simply become abstracted, as if unaware of his surroundings; on recovering consciousness, he would relate what he had seen, and learned, in his trance. More often – or perhaps it was more often reported, because it was more striking – he had what looked like a fit, foaming at the mouth and going into convulsions, until a voice sounding unlike his own would speak through him, or sometimes to him, as if he were the dummy of an invisible ventriloquist (it was to voices of this disembodied kind that the term 'ventriloquism' originally applied). His listeners' assumption was that he was possessed by a spirit, or spirits, who were using him as the agency by which they passed their information on to the tribe: warning, say, that a witch, or an evil spirit was at work, and recommending the appropriate remedies.

Sickness was attributed to a loss of soul-power. The sick person's soul or psyche, it was believed, was being abstracted by the spirits, or by a witch; the tribal doctor's function was to go in pursuit of it, and arrange for it to be returned. Another possibility was that a spirit or a witch had managed to materialise some malign substance in the patient's body; then, the tribal doctor would seek to remove it by de-materialising it, or by 'sucking it out'. Or he might put his patients into trances like his own, with the help of rhythm and drugs, inducing convulsions, dissociation, and eventually comas; the belief being that they too had been possessed by friendly spirits, helping to cure them.

Diagnosis and treatment, in other words, were assumed to work by magic, in the original sense of the term: by forces of the kind now called psychic or paranormal. A tribal doctor obtained and held his post by virtue of the belief that with the help of spirits he could perceive and influence people and objects at a distance. By the time European explorers and missionaries began to report primitive customs, however, the ability of tribal doctors even to enter a trance state had begun to decline. Often they had to perform consciously; and when they put their questions, they might have to rely on devices of various kinds to register the answers. Some of them used a pendulum, allowing the direction in which the 'bob' swung to tell them what the spirits had in mind; some held sticks, which became agitated when the questioner was growing 'warm', as if the spirits were grabbing at it, to show the enquiry was on the right lines; some peered into bowls of water, or crystals, in the hope of prompting second sight; some threw bones, and interpreted according to the pattern in which they fell.

Diagnosis and treatment, though, were beginning to become what observers regarded as rational, or at least pragmatic. To deal with everyday sickness most tribes had an extensive pharmacopeia of herbal remedies, and relied on individuals skilled in dealing with fractures and dislocations. Yet even here, the psychic element survived. Herbs might need to be found with the help of second sight, and administered with the assistance of a spell or incantation. The feeling remained, too, that any illness which did not follow a normal course, or respond to treatment, must be psychically-induced – particularly if the sufferer were an important member of the community. Psychological and psychic forces – the two were not kept distinct – continued to be considered as determining whether people fell ill, and whether they would recover. And the tribal doctor's influence continued to depend on his ability to convince the tribe of his powers as a diviner, witch-finder, and communicator of remedies prescribed by the spirits, rather than on his knowledge of herbs or other aids.

SHAMANISM IN DECLINE

The powers attributed to the shaman, medicine man or witch doctor, though, meant that he was not just the tribal doctor. He would also consult the spirits about whether the tribe should move camp, either to find game or to avoid a marauding enemy tribe. He might be credited with the power to bring rain, or divert storms. He was often, in effect, the tribe's legislator, with the chief as the executive. And this meant that when the early civilisations began to establish themselves, he could be a threat to the central authority. What happened as a result can be gauged from the course events were later to follow in the colonial era, from the time of the Spanish conquistadors on through to the dividing-up of equatorial Africa. Always, the shaman was regarded as subversive, because by virtue of his calling he regarded himself as above the law. But his magic was no match for the white man's bullets; he had to conform, or face imprisonment and execution. As a result, he lost ground to the tribal herbalist.

By the time of the early civilisations, Egypt and Babylon, the herbalists had come to be recognised as the technicians of medicine (their remedies including drugs: elaborate animal and mineral as well as vegetable compounds), and the shamans' functions had been divided up between the magicians and the priests. The 'magi' claimed psychic powers, but they had largely abandoned inspirational divination in favour of systematised techniques; more sophisticated versions of 'throwing the bones'. Omens were observed, and the entrails of sacrificial animals consulted. Some diviners may have used the entrails as many a palmist today uses the lines on the hand; not as a direct guide, but as a way of liberating intuition. But as elaborate charts were available it was possible for the Babylonian diviner simply to read off the diagnosis from the appearance and condition of the entrails, as a palm can now be read from a manual of instruction. And although treatment was accompanied by rites and incantations, these appear to have reflected a kind of insurance policy, like 'touching wood' today. The psychic element was subordinate except in connection with possession. The belief remained that convulsions represented possession by a spirit; but there was no longer confidence that the spirit's intentions were necessarily estimable. It might be good; it might be evil. Possession had become something to be feared; if menacing, to be exorcised by a priest.

Shamanism, however, made a last stand, graphically portrayed in the Old Testament. Even if it cannot be relied upon as a historical record of what happened, it can be trusted as a record of what was believed; and one belief, in particular, has left its mark on medicine. The shaman, or prophet, was often in communication with spirits – angels. But they were not acting in their own right. They were merely the messengers from a master-spirit – the Lord. And belief in the Lord – not, at first, as the only god, but to the Israelites, as the only *true* god – created a new attitude to disease which has influenced medicine to this day. The prophets no longer relied upon spontaneous or induced spirit promptings to tell them what to do for the sick. As the Lord was in sole charge of the destinies of the tribe and of each of its members, sickness could only be by his intent. And as sickness was unpleasant, he presumably intended it as a punishment; the only notable exception being Job, whom Satan was permitted to infect with boils from head to toe in order to test his fidelity.

There was consequently little point in the prophets, or anybody else, trying to cure illness. 'There is no god with me,' the Lord told Moses. 'I kill and I make alive; I wound, and I heal; neither is there any that can deliver out of my hand.' The prophets were rarely chronicled in their old shaman role as healers. It might, therefore, seem illogical that the Israelites should have introduced and rigorously enforced a set of regulations for diet and hygiene which marked the introduction of effective preventive medicine. Yet if it is accepted that the original role of the shamans had been to divine what the spirits (or instinct and intuition) were trying to communicate through the conscious mind's blockade, then it ceases to be surprising that Moses should have emphasised the necessity for such rules, while attributing them, as he attributed everything which he heard in his mind's ear, to the Lord.

The existence of a written sanitary code, coupled with the growing influence of the technicians – druggists and bonesetters – was gradually to create the division into what later were to be regarded as the vitalist and the mechanist schools. The basic vitalist belief, derived from the shaman era, was that psychological, psychic or spirit forces were responsible for making people ill, and had to be invoked to help them to recover. The mechanist belief was that people became ill because of, say, over-indulgence, or sitting around in damp clothes after being caught in the rain, and that they needed rest and a suitable diet. The two creeds were not entirely antagonistic: vitalists accepted that people who were poisoned would die, and mechanists conceded that the gods might intervene to cause illness. But their differences began to show in their methods of diagnosis and treatment.

HIPPOCRATES

To judge from Homer, the ancient Greeks had much the same attitude to disease as the Israelites, except that they believed it to be a punishment not so much for sinning as for offending one of the gods, or falling into the clutches of a sorceress. After Homer's time, however, the reputation of Aesculapius, a deified mortal, led to the emergence of a cult; he was worshipped for his special powers to heal diseases. The sick could come to his temples for purification, and in the hope of obtaining divine instruction while in a trance state, or in dreams. Miraculous cures were claimed – in all probability, Henry Sigerist argued in his *History of Medicine*, with justification; it was easy to imagine the patient's state of mind 'when the great moment, long anticipated with hope and awe, had arrived, when he was going to face his living god. In such moments of great nervous tension miracles do occur, or at least happenings which are difficult to explain.

But the cult had a rival. Having established themselves in Greece as practitioners in their own right, by the fifth century B.C. medical technicians were recognisably physicians. One of them was Hippocrates of Cos; a number of treatises attributed to him have survived, though it is not possible to be sure which, if any, of them he actually wrote. They give a remarkably clear picture of the theories, practices and attitudes of Greek medicine at the time, covering diagnosis and prognosis, physiology and pathology, prevention and treatment.

The Hippocratic school did not reject vitalism so much as set it to one side. What Fate had in store – what the gods or the spirits might be up to – was the individual's private concern; for the physician, the most important thing was to treat disease as and when it arose, and this prompted speculation about how and why it arose. It might be due to external influences, such as climate, or to internal influences, such as over-indulgence; but always it could be traced to specific

causes. The symptoms of sore throat, say, or influenza – the
writer of the treatise on tradition in medicine insisted – were
caused simply by 'the presence of certain substances which,
when present, invariably produce such results' – the earliest
surviving presentation of the mechanistic case.

One of the writers went further. 'I do not believe,' his
treatise began, 'that the Sacred Disease is any more divine or
sacred than any other disease but, on the contrary, has
specific characteristics and a definite cause.' The 'sacred disease' was epilepsy; but the term had a wider connotation,
including hysteria and possession. In Homer's time, it had
been assumed that possession was 'sacred' in the sense that the
gods were very ready to enter mortals when it suited their
purposes; but by the fifth century the gods were no longer
expected to play such tricks. People often went out of their
minds, doing strange things like shouting in their sleep, or
even sleep-walking, the Hippocratic writer observed; and nobody suggested there was anything 'sacred' about such symptoms. Those who called fits sacred, he believed, 'were the sort
of people we now call witch-doctors, quacks, and charlatans',
who were invoking a divine element to hide their inability to
provide effective medical treatment.

Although the Hippocratic school's insistence that epilepsy
was not divine has generally been regarded as a step in the
direction of more rational attitudes to health and disease, it
also led to the rejection of the possibility that dissociation
and convulsions could be a useful therapeutic aid. Yet ironically Hippocrates' contemporary, Socrates, described how he
himself had benefited throughout his life from the ability to
dissociate, and hear a spirit voice. He would not contest the
death sentence, he told his judges, because what he regarded
as a divine faculty, the voice in his mind's ear which guided
him in all he did, had not intervened. This guidance, he believed, emanated from his 'daemon' – his guardian angel. It
had always warned him if he were about to do anything of
which it disapproved; or he could enter a trance state to consult it – as presumably he did, or could do, about his health.

The repudiation of inspirational diagnosis and treatment
would have mattered less if all physicians had been able

to maintain the Hippocratic school's cautious pragmatism. But even in its treatises there were signs of a craving for a new philosophy of medicine based on a material, rather than spiritist, principle; and this led to the acceptance of the idea that disease is the consequence of some imbalance in the body's 'humours'.

The theory had originated in India, but had been distorted in its travels: the Greeks held that there were four, not three, humours; and their composition was different, blood, phlegm, black bile and yellow bile. If the proportions were correct, the assumption was that the individual would be healthy: ill-health indicated a need to restore the balance between them. The 'balance' principle was not substantially different from Claude Bernard's theory of the body's self-regulatory mechanism, on which present-day physiology is largely based; but the practice which was derived from it was 'allopathy' – the use of medicines designed to counteract symptoms in order to redress the balance; and as a consequence mechanistic medicine became identified with allopathic remedies.

The remedies were often horrendous; particularly after Galen had made his reputation as physician to Marcus Aurelius in the second century A.D. Ostensibly of the Hippocratic school, he was to subvert its saner teachings. Hippocrates, Galen admitted, had led the way. But he had not followed it up. 'He opened the road, I have made it passable.' As royal physician Galen was able to impose his views on how the road should be followed; and as a prolific writer, he saw to it that they were publicised. They included enthusiastic approval for treatment with drugs, and in particular by combinations of drugs. The drugs of the time were a mixture of traditional herbal remedies with more esoteric animal and mineral innovations: powdered rhinoceros horn; dried camel dung; precious metals, mixed or compounded according to the whim of the doctor. And some of Galen's prescriptions required a hundred or more different substances, all justified with reference to the humours: 'as cool as a cucumber' derives from his faith in that vegetable as the drug of choice when, in his opinion, the imbalance was due to excessive heat.

All that Rome had to offer in the advancement of medicine, in fact, was a renewed dedication to hygiene, and in particular to the provision of abundant supplies of pure drinking water (whether hot baths were popular because, as Pliny claimed, steam from hot springs had been found to be wholesome and good for rheumatism and ulcers or whether, as Horace believed, it was simply from self-indulgence, remains a matter of opinion).

CHRISTIAN HEALING

In the absence of any recognised vitalist therapy magic began to re-emerge in self-medication, with the use of charms and incantations to supplement folklore remedies; but as described by Pliny in his *Natural History*, debased by superstition. When vitalism recovered it was through the impact of Christianity. Jesus's teachings differed from those of the earlier prophets in one significant respect: his instructions from the Lord were to heal the sick. Although the assumption remained that they were sick because of their sins or loss of faith, Jesus believed he could offer instant cures – 'thy sins be forgiven thee'; 'thy faith hath made thee whole' – to those who repented. Given the restoration of the soul in an unblemished condition, the body – the expectation was – could also instantly be restored, even in cases of leprosy.

Jesus restored inspirational healing to respectability. It no longer had to be regarded as a waste of time because God had ordained the illness. On the contrary, it was a way of bringing lost souls back to God. And Jesus offered more; he made it clear to the disciples that they, too, could enjoy healing powers, a promise redeemed at Pentecost, when they believed they were possessed by God – by the Holy Spirit. They dissociated in traditional shaman fashion, losing control of their limbs, and speaking in strange tongues; and they found they were endowed with powers to heal the sick.

For the early Christians healing became as important a part of their mission as it had been to Jesus. They assumed it was a divine force which, through their possession by the Holy Spirit, they were able to transmit to suitable recipients; or which they could use to counter witchcraft, as Paul did when he struck the false prophet, Bar-Jesus, blind. For Paul, in parti-cular, Christianity was essentially inspirational. The spirit must be allowed to manifest itself, he insisted in his first epistle to the Corinthians. To one man might be given wis-dom, 'to another faith, by the same spirit; to another the gifts of healing, by the same spirit'. And pentecostal fervour was to suffuse and sustain Christianity throughout the long years of persecution under the Roman Empire, until at last Christians were rewarded by the authorities' recognition of, and con-version to, their faith.

No sooner had their faith become an established religion, however, than pentecostalism went the way of shamanism. For two centuries after the crucifixion Christians relied on in-spiration and miracle-working to guide them; but prophesy-ing, healing and other by-products of dissociation became un-welcome when, as they so often did, they appeared to promote what the Church leaders regarded as heresy. 'Covet to prophesy,' Paul had urged, 'and forbid not to speak with tongues.' But his advice 'let all things be done decently and with order' provided the excuse to dispense with prophesying, as the dissemination of heresy threatened church discipline. Possession, too, became suspect; it might be Satan, craftily passing himself off as the Holy Spirit.

Trance healing suffered from guilt by association; and in the Middle Ages the Church gradually backed out of its heal-ing mission. Later, in their drive against heresy, the Church's Inquisitors found that an easy way to justify what they were doing was to accuse suspects of practising witchcraft; this put the surviving purveyors of the magical element in folk medi-cine, spells and incantations, at risk. And although the Church approved of hospitals for the poor, at the Council of Tours in the twelfth century Pope Alexander III warned that the devil was seducing clergy to treat the sick with the excuse that they were serving suffering humanity. The study of medicine, the Pope feared, submitted them to many mundane temptations; in future treatment was to be left to the physicians.

With the Vatican becoming increasingly involved in tem-poral matters the way was open for physicians to establish themselves as, in effect, a craft guild; and in 1224 the Emperor Frederick II issued an ordinance laying down that nobody in future would be allowed to style himself a doctor unless he had passed a qualifying examination to obtain a licence. Regulations were also made for the practice of surgery. To the physician, surgeons were upstart artisans – carpenters, who happened to work on the human body rather than in wood. But many of them practised as tooth-pullers, stitchers-up of severe cuts and barbers, activities which could not be suppressed. In wars, too, particularly in the Hundred Years' War, they became indispensable. From time to time attempts were made by warrior monarchs to settle the difference between them and the physicians, and following Agincourt Henry V tried to bring them together; but a College of Medicine and Surgery set up in 1423 soon foundered. Relations between those surgeons who regarded themselves simply as surgeons and those who worked as barbers were also often strained; but their mutual resentment at the attitude of the physicians was eventually to bring them together to set up a separate Guild.

At the close of the Middle Ages, diagnosis and treatment of the sick – for those who could afford it – were largely in the hands of the physicians, still dedicated followers of Galen, relying more and more on 'polypharmacy', prescribing ever more complex compounds ('The more benumbed creative thought,' Sigerist observed, 'the larger is the space occupied by drugs'), purging, and blood-letting. Vitalism had sunk almost out of sight. Even nature's cures had been debased. Where the establishments founded by the Romans to exploit local sources of water had survived, or had been revived, their reputation was hardly above today's massage parlours; the Bishop of Bath and Wells complained in the mid-fifteenth century that respectable women taking the waters were abused and even fined if, from modesty, they refused to strip. Natural medicine was practised mainly by quacks in the cities and by village crones in the countryside; and in the case of the crones, practised at the risk of being charged with witchcraft, and burned at the stake.

Chapter Two

THE RENAISSANCE

The Renaissance gave the opportunity for doctors – and their critics – to re-examine Galenism; and one of the initial reactions was a revival of vitalist ideas, largely derived from alchemy. Though primarily chemists the alchemists had worked on the assumption that there were unexplained forces which, if they could be harnessed, could be used not just to turn base metals into gold, or provide an elixir of youth (these were the 'come-ons', to attract patronage and funds), but also to re-discover the powers, including healing, which shamans had been able to exercise.

ALCHEMISTS AND RATIONALISTS

Why – Cornelius Agrippa asked in his treatise on occult philosophy, published in 1531 – should magic and miracles, accepted unquestioningly by the early Church, have fallen into disrepute? He proposed to vindicate magic, so that it could be 'studied by all the wise, purged and free from the errors of impiety, and adorned with its own reasonable system'. Paracelsus agreed. The mind, he believed, could transcend its normal powers when trained to do so, for various purposes, healing among them.

Paracelsus rejected Galenism, and although he accepted the wisdom of the Hippocratic school's reliance upon nature's healing force he believed that the force contained magic elements of a kind whose significance the school had not realized. The effectiveness of herbal remedies, too, could be increased by techniques calculated to foster belief in them: the imagination could be so strengthened by faith that it could work what appeared to be miracles. Miracles were not superstitious nonsense, as rationalists were claiming; it was a credulous attitude to them which was superstitious. Witches did not fly to Sabbats to kiss the devil's rump, nor did they practise black magic. In magic there was no black and white: the distinction was between magic employed to give power over people, and magic employed to give power *for* people, as in healing.

Paracelsus's denunciations of Galen, and the often intemperate way in which he made them, made him unpopular with orthodox physicians; and the Church was in no mood to welcome a revival of magical practices associated with heresy and paganism. He was dismissed as a charlatan. But another threat to the Church was to prove more dangerous: rationalism. Vesalius's *On the Structure of the Human Body*, ostensibly a treatise describing what had been learned from the dissection of cadavers, amounted to a manifesto on behalf of rationalist science: a demand that the results of research should no longer be twisted to fit accepted religious or Galenic doctrines, however venerable. Along with Copernicus, whose treatise nominating the sun as the centre of the planetary system also appeared in 1543, Vesalius was launching the scientific revolution.

For the next hundred years the revolutionaries could follow either Paracelsus or Vesalius. Some of the greatest of them followed both; Van Helmont, Boyle and Newton were alchemists. But their researches failed to penetrate alchemy's secrets; and ironically, their contributions to science hastened the process by which alchemy was discredited. If so much of what had previously been inexplicable could now be explained without invoking the existence of the 'supernatural' – the term was just coming into use to describe anything which could not be fitted into the new framework of the 'laws' of nature – science would surely eventually be able to explain everything naturally, and rationally; including, of course, disease.

Scientific rationalism completed the process begun in the Middle Ages of severing the Church from medicine. Although priests continued to attend patients who were parishioners, such visits tended to be only for spiritual consolation. Divine healing was acceptable only when it occurred, or could be claimed as having occurred, through the intervention of the Blessed Virgin or of some Christian martyr. Cures were occasionally claimed for priests, monks or nuns during their lifetime; but the Vatican was by this time reluctant to accept as divine any miracle which might encourage the sin of pride. Death was the great levitator; anybody from whose shrine miraculous cures were reported stood a chance of beatification, and eventually canonisation – though to protect itself, the Vatican employed a 'devil's advocate', to put the case against accepting the cures as miraculous. The role was taken seriously; it was not in the Church's interest to accept miracles whose spurious nature might later be exposed, to the delight of its adversaries.

The Protestant attitude to healing moved even further away from that of the early Christians. By the seventeenth century, Keith Thomas has noted in his *Religion and the Decline of Magic*, prayer was designed to supplement treatment, not to supersede it. Miracles were regarded as 'the swaddling bands of the early Church, necessary for the initial conversion of unbelievers, but redundant once the faith had securely established itself'. Healing was practised by pentecostal sects, such as the Quakers originally were; and the belief in divine intervention lingered on in 'touching for the King's evil'. But Church of England clergy came to regard the laying-on of hands as no more than a ritual gesture, accompanying a prayer for the sick.

By the seventeenth century, such vitalist beliefs and practices as remained were to be found chiefly among the poor, and although every town and village had its 'cunning man' or 'wise woman' dispensing herbs and magical remedies, they were still at risk of being charged with witchcraft if these did not work, or worked too explosively. And natural medicine also suffered in another way; one of the consequences of the split between science and the supernatural was the decline of herbalism.

Many beliefs had attached themselves to herbs: that those which resembled human features would be useful in the treatment of those features (a plant with a flower shaped like an ear, say, for earache); that they should be picked in accordance with astrological signs, or at certain times of day; and that certain incantations should accompany the processes by which they were made into medicines. Following the Renaissance herbalists were torn between a desire to get rid of what they felt to be the barnacles of old superstition, in order to put their craft on a rational basis, and the feeling that perhaps the magical tradition was, or would be shown to be, scientific. In his *History of Plants*, published towards the end of Queen Elizabeth I's reign, John Gerard insisted that his recipes were 'not for the use of the beggarly rabble of witches, charmers and such-like': the virtue of the plant medicines, he believed, resided in the plants and not in the ceremonial attached to harvesting them. But to Culpeper, half a century later, it seemed obvious that as plants reacted to moisture, light and heat they were as subject to planetary influences as people; the herbalist must consequently be an astrologer. And Culpeper's *Pharmacopeia*, written in English instead of the Latin which doctors and scientists still favoured, linked herbalism firmly in the public mind with astrology – just at the time when astrology was falling into scientific disfavour.

So long as Galenic polypharmacy remained fashionable, too, faith in the efficacy of remedies made up from single herbs seemed naïve. The herbalists still relied chiefly on 'simples', each herb being believed to be a remedy for some specific symptom. But in that case, physicians felt, it would surely be sensible to use compounds designed to clear up all the symptoms, as a sick person often had several at once: headache, sore throat, running nose, fever. Druggists in their own interest naturally advocated this course; and the word 'simple' came to be used in its familiar contemptuous sense.

Physicians and druggists – they were now styling themselves apothecaries – catered for the wealthy and their retainers; and although Paracelsus and Vesalius had both, in their different ways, discredited Galen, Galenism remained the accepted orthodoxy. In *Le Malade Imaginaire* Argan was able to satisfy his examiners by repeating the same prescription for each disease – enemas, bleeding, purging; and when asked what he would do if this treatment failed, by telling them that he would recommend another enema, more bleeding, and more purging. And that this was not simply Molière's fantasy was to be agonisingly demonstrated twelve years later, when King Charles II fell ill with a kidney complaint.

In *The Last Days of Charles II* Raymond Crawfurd, drawing on contemporary sources (including a number of eye-witness accounts) was able to give an hour-by-hour account of the tortures to which the King was subjected. First, sixteen ounces of blood were removed from his right arm by a surgeon. When the physicians arrived 'they ordered cupping glasses to be applied to his shoulders forthwith, and deep scarification to be carried out, by which they succeeded in removing another eight ounces'. A strong antimonial emetic was administered; as he could not swallow all of it 'they determined to render assurance doubly sure by a full dose of Sulphate of Zinc', along with purgatives, a succession of clysters, and cantharides (the blistering agent, 'Spanish fly') applied to his shorn head. 'As though this was not enough, the red-hot cautery was requisitioned as well.' For four days and nights fourteen physicians vied with each other to prescribe these and other remedies, including Peruvian bark, increasing quantities of Sal Ammoniac, and various products of poly-pharmacy. Eventually 'the Oriental Bezoar Stone, from its normal habitat in the stomach of an eastern goat, was transferred to its last resting place in that of the king'. Charles apologised to those around him for being such 'an unconscionable time a-dying'; it is hard not to assume that they precipitated his death.

SYDENHAM

Many poor people, as Thomas Sydenham had observed, must have owed their lives to the fact that they could not afford medical treatment. Sydenham was the outstanding medical thinker of his time, not from any profound originality, but from a combination of humility, integrity and commonsense. His *Treatise on Fevers*, published in 1666, represented a return to the approach of the Hippocratic school, which he revered. It was also, in effect, a denunciation of medicine as practised by members of the College of Physicians (the Royal College, as it was soon to become). Membership was confined to 'learned and weighty men', which in practice meant that they had learned medicine by studying Greek and Latin texts at a university; as Sydenham put it 'One might as well send a man to Oxford to learn shoe-making as practising physic.' The only place to study medicine, he insisted, was at the bed-side, learning how to diagnose what was the matter with patients, and how to treat them. There was not very much a doctor could do, he admitted. A few simples and a few drugs could help; otherwise, it was chiefly a matter of throwing out the accumulated Galenic rubbish, and relying on nature's healing powers.

Sydenham, though, had another point to make: that symptoms ought to be more clearly distinguished from diseases. A headache was a symptom; but it might have many causes, from influenza to over-indulgence in alcohol. The doctor's aim, therefore, should be to look behind the symptom, and diagnose the cause. And eminently sensible though this advice was, it provided the orthodox physicians of the type he despised with a new weapon. The ability to diagnose the source (or what was believed to be the source) of symptoms, and to give it a name, would reassure as well as impress patients, even if treatments were as disastrous as ever.

French doctors, in particular, were attracted to the new 'nosology' – the science of classifying diseases in the way that Linnaeus was classifying plants; and in the middle of the eighteenth century Boissier de Sauvages' massive treatise on nosology revealed the effect the new science was having: creating the impression that diseases existed in their own right, as physical entities. Descartes' dualism, the doctrine that mind and matter exist as independent entities, made it pos-sible to put body and spirit in separate compartments; and the flood of new discoveries about the body, notably those of Newton and Malpighi about the circulation of the blood, and of Borelli about the neurological links between brain and muscle, encouraged the belief that illness would eventually be explained on straightforward physiological principles. Borelli went further, claiming that it would be explained on straightforward *mechanical* principles. By the nineteenth century the mechanists, as by this time they were beginning to call themselves, had virtually eliminated spiritual, psychic and psychological forces from their calculations.

Sydenham's teachings had appeared to have one immediately beneficial effect: the new-style medical school founded in Holland by Boerhaave, where the teaching was in the vernacular – and in a clinic, around the patients' beds. Soon students were flocking to Leyden from all over Europe; and similar establishments began to open up in many cities linked with, but no longer entirely subordinate to, the universities. But these, the forerunners of the teaching hospitals, actually strengthened the physicians' control over medical practice, as the Decrees of Marly, promulgated by Louis XIV in 1707, foreshadowed. They laid down that medicine was only to be taught in recognised schools; that a minimum three years of training, with periodic examinations, would be required before any student could qualify as a doctor; and that 'No person may practise medicine, or prescribe any remedy, even without payment, if he has not obtained the degree.' Although the authorities were to find it difficult to restrict medical training in this way, and impossible to prevent unqualified practitioners from practising, the decrees reflected the view that the State had a duty to protect citizens from exploitation by charlatans and quacks; and it was the physicians who were expected to provide the trained and qualified alternative. Where a government was strong and efficient enough, therefore, the physicians could expect to enjoy professional and monopoly status; and this increased the pressure on students to accept whatever principles and practices were taught at the time.

ST MEDARD

By the eighteenth century, therefore, mechanism was taking a firm hold: so firm that it was unshaken even by the extraordinary episode of the *convulsionnaires* of St Médard. In the late 1720's the tomb of François de Paris became a place of pilgrimage to which the sick began to arrive in great numbers, seeking cures. The process was usually accompanied by convulsions, dissociation and other pentecostal phenomena; and what happened was well-documented, witnessed as it was by many distinguished visitors who came as sceptics, but were convinced by what they saw. Even more remarkable than the cures were the numerous reports, also well-attested, of individuals who in their ecstatic states were able to demonstrate that they could be slashed at, pounded with heavy mallets, or roasted over fires, without suffering injury or pain.

The St Médard manifestations continued for the best part of a decade; and the accumulated evidence impressed even Diderot, who had to admit it challenged the scepticism 'of the most stubborn'. But by this time the medical profession, having turned its back in what it regarded as superstition, was not prepared to jeopardise its new-found principles by trying to fit convulsions and incombustibility into them. Such things, the feeling was, had not happened because they could not have happened; they were against the laws of nature. In his essay on miracles David Hume was actually to use St Médard in support of his scepticism. The miracles, he admitted, had been 'proved upon the spot by judges of unquestioned integrity, attested by witnesses of credit', and had never been refuted. But this, for him, simply illustrated the fact that not even the most meticulously documented and witnessed report could be trusted, if what was reported did not square with nature's laws.

In different circumstances the Catholic Church might have been tempted to try to exploit St Médard to resume its healing mission. But François de Paris had been a member of the quasi-Calvinist sect of Jansenists, whose beliefs and activities were unpopular in Rome; and the need to explain the miracles away was probably one of the reasons which prompted Prosper Lambertini, the future Pope Benedict XIV, to write a treatise which was to de-fuse the controversy within the Church, and also to define the Church's attitude.

Lambertini had for a time been devil's advocate; he was well acquainted with the problems, and he laid down a rigorous set of conditions. A cure could be considered as divinely miraculous if the disease was of a kind known to be hard to cure; if the possibility of spontaneous remission could be ruled out; if earlier medical treatment had been unsuccessful; if the cure was immediate, or at least came very soon after intercession; if the cure was complete; if it could not be regarded as the consequence of the overcoming of some natural crisis; if there was no relapse; and if the patient remained well, no other disease developing. Of these, only the last was to become inoperative, presumably because it was thought to be too stringent.

Lambertini was humane as well as shrewd, as his biographer Renée Haynes has shown; and the fact that his conditions have survived almost unchanged to the present day reflects how far ahead his thinking was of his time. But he was also a man of his time; and of his faith. To Catholics convulsions were associated with the devil. It seemed inconceivable that the St Médard happenings could be the work of God. And in order to play down St Médard, Lambertini had to invoke mass hysteria, quoting Sydenham to the effect that 'Proteus hath no more shapes, nor the chameleon so great a variety of colours' – the implication being that emotional contagion could account for what otherwise would seem inexplicable in natural terms. If hysteria could not merely save people from feeling pain when subjected to assault with mallets, knives and fire, but also permit them to emerge apparently unscathed, then it deserved investigating in its own right, to find out how; but this was not what Lambertini wanted.

FOLK MEDICINE

With the Church abstaining, and orthodox medicine catering only for the minority who could afford physicians' fees and the cost of the drugs they prescribed, the general public had had to continue to rely on self-medication reinforced by folk medicine; and it was only rarely that such practices, and their practitioners, attracted attention. Ordinary fractures or dislocated joints, for example, were usually taken to the local bonesetter, particularly as they so often occurred in the country, in riding accidents; and the bonesetter was on much the same social and educational level as the 'cunning man' –

a farm-worker, perhaps, or an artisan who had taken to manipulation either because he had a knack for it or because the techniques were passed down from father to son.

Naturally bonesetters did not often have a reputation outside the locality in which they worked; but one exception was Sarah Mapp, a Surrey woman who was featured in an article in the *London Magazine* in 1736, (and also in one of Hogarth's cartoons, purporting to display the coat of arms of the 'Company of Undertakers'). Mrs Mapp made her name by dealing expeditiously with dislocations and fractures which had baffled fashionable London surgeons, so that she drew clients from the aristocracy, even from royalty. The story was told about her that when some surgeons, anxious to expose her as a quack, sent her a patient telling him to pretend his wrist was out of joint, she promptly put it out of joint, telling him to go back 'to the fools who sent him, and get it set again'. Sarah Mapp's skill, though, was not of a kind which could readily be taught; and the largely uneducated bonesetters could not hope to establish an organisation. So although a doctor, particularly a country doctor, would no more have hesitated to send patients to the local bonesetter than he would now hesitate to take his car for repairs to the local garage, bonesetting continued to be regarded as set apart from medicine.

Medicine was also, by this time, set apart from magic; as folk medicine was also coming to be. 'Cunning men' and 'wise women' were still to be found in most villages; but the development of natural cures divorced from magic was reflected in John Wesley's *Primitive Physick*, published in 1768. Wesley might have been expected to stress the spiritual aspects of health, and he did; but he also showed that he believed in nature's remedies in their own right.

God, Wesley argued, created man incorruptible and immortal. 'As he knew no sin, so he knew no pain, no sickness, weakness or bodily disorder.' There should consequently be no place for physic, or the art of healing; partly because if a man led a good life, nature would supply all that he needed for good health; but also because, as Sydenham and Boerhaave had shown, compounded drugs not merely lost the power of simples, but could 'commence a strong and deadly poison'. To preserve or regain health Wesley recommended a plain diet, with no highly seasoned food; water, or 'good, clear small-beer'; regular exercise: and early-to-bed-and-early-to-rise. These, he felt, could be more than half the cure. And though he recommended faith and prayer, he clearly thought of them as essential for their own sake; and not as ritual accompaniment of the remedies he recommended for particular disorders.

Herbalism, too, was gradually being stripped of its associations with astrology and magic; and this made it easier for orthodoxy to appropriate its ideas, in the way it did following the publication of William Withering's *Account of the Foxglove* in 1785. Withering had made his name ten years earlier with a botanical work describing British vegetables; but he had had little to say about their medicinal properties because, as he put it, 'those who are best enabled to judge of the matter will perhaps think that the greater part of that little might well have been omitted' – typical of orthodoxy's attitude. He shared Sydenham's and Boerhaave's mistrust, however, of the still prevailing fashion of polypharmacy: 'Combining a great variety of ingredients with a design to answer any particular purpose rendered the efficacy of any of them extremely doubtful.' And this had prompted him to research into simples, so that while 'rejecting the fables of the ancient herbalist', he could re-assess their values 'on the basis of accurate and well-considered experiments'.

An opportunity for experiment had presented itself as a result of awaiting a change of horses at a Staffordshire inn. Asked to treat a woman with dropsy he had decided that she was unlikely to survive; but when he next passed that way he was surprised to find she had recovered as the result, it was claimed, of drinking a herbal tea. Investigating, he came to the conclusion that the plant responsible must be the foxglove; he proceeded to test his hypothesis on one hundred and sixty three patients; and his conclusion was that the drug from the plant, digitalis, was more effective and less toxic in the treatment of heart conditions and associated symptoms, such as dropsy, than any of the remedies then in standard use.

But the credit for the discovery went not to the herbalists, or to traditional medicine, but to Withering; and the physicians enjoyed their colleague's reflected glory.

THE 'STROKERS'

The only remaining chance for natural medicine to stage a recovery was through dissensions arising among the physicians, or from some demonstration of vitalism which they could not reject. But when such demonstrations were presented they were never quite convincing enough. Only one individual came close to proving the reality of natural – or, as he preferred to believe, divine – healing: Valentine Greatrakes.

Although Greatrakes had fought for Cromwell he had managed to avoid Royalist retribution after the restoration of the monarchy; and back on his Irish estate he found that if he went through the motions of the laying-on of hands (or of 'stroking' people who were ill, without actually touching them: they did not need to remove their clothes), their symptoms – tumours, paralysis, deafness, headaches, arthritis – often disappeared.

As a popular member of the Anglo-Irish society, a landowner and a magistrate, Greatrakes could demonstrate his powers to neighbours, including peers and bishops, without being accused of witchcraft. Such a healing force, he was careful to reassure them, could only come from God. He was also able to convince Boyle and another member of the Royal Society, John Wilkins, that his cures were genuine. In 1666 – the year of the publication of Sydenham's treatise on fevers – Greatrakes arrived in England on what turned out to be a spectacular healing tour; and he published an account of his methods, with detailed case histories, such as the cure of Eleanor Dickinson, a dropsy sufferer for twelve years. After his laying-on of hands she had felt a rumbling in her belly, 'and brake great stores of wind *per anum et per partem domesticam*' before making water copiously, several gallons in the next twenty-four hours, until her belly was 'as empty as a glove or purse, and wraps over'.

Inevitably there were accusations of fraud; but in view of the fact that he freely admitted his method did not work consistently (it failed when he gave a demonstration before Charles II), and that he refused payment for his services, no really damaging revelations were produced to set off against the range of reported cures and the standing of the witnesses who attested them. But if Greatrakes could not easily be discredited, the physicians had another weapon. They could ignore 'stroking', just as they politely ignored 'touching for the king's evil'. Greatrakes retired to his estate, and was soon forgotten.

Some of the people Greatrakes cured exhibited the symptoms traditionally associated with tribal healing – or, as it had later become when adopted by priests, with exorcism. In the middle of the eighteenth century a Swiss priest who had been cured by exorcism of a mental disorder began to practise it himself; and his patients often reacted in the traditional way, going into convulsions, dissociating, talking in strange voices and eventually falling into comas. His cures of physical as well as of mental disorders were attested by many reliable witnesses, who also emphasised Gassner's dedication to his faith, and his refusal to allow himself to be affected by the malice of those who condemned him, often unseen, as a charlatan. But the Vatican, still under Lambertini's influence – he lived on until 1758 – was not willing to accept that cures of this kind, too reminiscent of St Médard, were divine. It would be in the church's interest, though, if they were not divine, to trace them to some mundane source. Fr Hehl, S J, Professor of Astronomy at the University of Vienna, began to experiment to see if some rational explanation for the phenomena might be found; and he tried using magnets, to see if they would make any difference.

Paracelsus had suggested that magnetism might be one of the ways in which human beings were inter-connected, even at a distance; Van Helmont had thought that everybody was susceptible to it; and for a while in the early seventeenth century a controversy had been stirred up on the issue, clerical writers vehemently denouncing the idea, fearing that it was just another insidious attempt to account for divine intervention in rational terms. Now, in a sense, the Vatican was on the same side as the scientists. Magnetism might be invoked to explain away St Médard. Aspiring scientists were also intrigued; and among those who came to witness Hehl's experiments was a graduate of the university, Franz Mesmer.

MESMERISM

Mesmer had become interested in the subject as a student; in the dissertation he was called upon to give when he graduated in 1766 he had chosen to propound the thesis that a 'subtle fluid' pervaded the universe, much as gravity did, which influenced people as the moon influenced the tides. From experiments he found that by advancing or withdrawing a magnet he could influence the rate of the flow of blood from a patient who was being bled. But he also found that it was not necessary to use the magnet. The influence could be transmitted by any object he had 'magnetised' by 'stroking' it; or simply by pointing his forefinger much as a shaman might do 'pointing the bone'. As in Gassner's exorcisms Mesmer's patients often went into convulsions, trances, and comas; and they also felt much the better for the treatment. Magnetism, Mesmer believed, was the explanation, but it was *animal* magnetism; a force from space, or from the planets, capable of being transmitted through people, which could act upon living organisms independently of actual metal magnets.

The Austrian physicians had not felt seriously threatened by Gassner or Hehl; but the vogue animal magnetism began to enjoy disturbed them, and Mesmer was driven from Vienna. Finding his way to Paris he again attracted a devoted following; and again encountered the same violent and often unscrupulous opposition. He had been fortunate enough to win friends at court, and in 1784 Louis XVI called for an enquiry by members of the Academies of the Sciences and of Medicine to test his claims. Correctly assuming that so many of the Academicians were so implacably hostile that he would not get a fair trial Mesmer declined to co-operate; but his disciple D'Eslon stood in for him in what was the most elaborate investigation yet made of a clinical technique.

D'Eslon's treatment consisted of a combination of the laying-on of hands, 'stroking', and magnetism, the patients holding objects which had been previously 'magnetised'. The patients often went into convulsions, characterised by involuntary, jerking movements of the arms and legs, twitching, eyeball rollings, cries, strange noises and hysterical laughter. There could be no question of collusion, as had been suggested; the investigators had to admit the patients really were under the control of the magnetiser – D'Eslon. Nor did they dispute that patients were often cured of their symptoms by the use of the technique. But convulsions might be dangerous; in any case, what they had been called upon to investigate was not whether the method produced cures but whether, if it did, the cures were produced by animal magnetism. Their answer was an unequivocal negative. It was imagination, they decided, which was responsible for the cures. Animal magnetism 'being non-existent can have no salubrious effects'.

The commissioners were distinguished. They included Benjamin Franklin, as Chairman : Lavoisier; the great botanist Jussieu; the historian of astronomy, Bailly; and Guillotin, the inventor of the humane killer which still bears his name. But as Mesmer had feared, they brought their preconceptions to their task. It was not the first time that scientists had demonstrated their inability to set preconceptions aside; Lavoisier had earlier been one of a committee which had rejected evidence for the existence of meteorites, on the ground that the existence of meteorites was contrary to natural laws. But their reports also showed that they were capable of ignoring any evidence which did not fit their preconceptions. Patients occasionally reacted to a gesture from the magnetiser, Jussieu had observed, even when they could not see him. It followed, he felt, that some force other than the imagination must be involved. He was no more inclined than his colleagues to accept Mesmer's hypothesis; but he was honest enough to argue, in a minority report, that there must be some unexplained force 'which is exercised by man on man'. In their determination to discredit animal magnetism, however, the other commissioners rejected his finding.

Whether or not their condemnation would have sufficed

to destroy Mesmer's reputation was not to be tested; his links with the Court of Louis XVI were in themselves sufficient to damn him, after 1789, in the eyes of the revolutionaries – among them Bailly, destined to become President of the National Assembly, and Mayor of Paris, before perishing on the guillotine during the Terror. The same fate overtook Lavoisier, and would doubtless have claimed Mesmer, had he not already left France to become for a while a wanderer, before settling down to practise in Switzerland until his death in quiet obscurity. To dabble in animal magnetism had become hazardous, and was to remain so until the Bourbons were restored.

The revolution also provided the first indication that Jacobinism posed no threat to mechanistic orthodoxy. Physicians or surgeons might be at risk because of their political views or their aristocratic connections, but not because they were members of what by this time was recognisably a profession. The frequently expressed aim of the revolutionaries was to ensure that everybody had access to the kind of medical treatment that previously had been restricted to the aristocrats and the wealthier bourgeoisie, and by implication this meant that the kind of treatment the physicians and surgeons provided was regarded as worth having, a sentiment they were naturally willing to encourage. Revolutionaries of all shades, too, believing as they did that social and economic measures to improve the condition of the masses would also improve their health, tended to be mechanist in their attitudes; and this tied in with their suspicions of vitalism because of its associations with the Church.

In different circumstances the physicians and surgeons would have been alarmed at the numerous proposals to increase the powers of the State to promote health and to control disease; but as they themselves were to be allowed to wield the powers on the State's behalf – even, it was planned, to be allowed to control what textbooks should be published, and what treatments permitted, with special Health Courts to enforce their regulations – they were not disposed to resist.

The French Revolution and its aftermath, Foucault has observed in *The Birth of the Clinic*, saw the start of two great myths: 'The myth of a nationalised medical profession, organised like the clergy, and invested at the level of man's bodily health with powers similar to those exercised by the clergy over men's souls; and the myth of a total disappearance of disease in an untroubled dispassionate society, restored to its original state of health.' Although the revolutionary fervour did not last, physicians were happy to continue to foster the myths even after the Bourbon restoration, in the hope of consolidating their professional status and at the same time completing the transformation of medicine into a science finally liberated from superstition. By this time, however, they had another threat to their peace of mind and to their purses: homeopathy.

HOMEOPATHY

Samuel Hahnemann, of Meissen in Saxony, had qualified as a doctor in the ordinary way, but his interests from the start of his career had been wide-ranging; he was the translator of many scientific works into German, and a researcher into the chemistry of toxic drugs (becoming a friend of Lavoisier in that capacity). At the time he began to practise physicians all over Europe were attracted to the ideas expounded by John Brown in Edinburgh, and Broussais in Paris. All disorders, Brown believed, were due to an excess of stimulation. 'Sthenics', who suffered from the excess, should be treated by bleeding and sedatives; 'asthenics', those who were lacking, by stimulants. Broussais's idea was even simpler: all diseases were symptomatic of gastro-enteritis, so they could all be dealt with by massive bleedings and purgings. Appalled by their influence, and dissatisfied with allopathic theory, Hahnemann had begun to cast around for an alternative; and he found it in 1790, following some research he did into the effects of quinine.

'Peruvian bark', from which quinine had been derived, had been used by South American tribes to treat malaria, and had been adopted for the same purpose in Europe, the standard explanation being that it must be an antidote. Hahnemann, experimenting on himself, found that quinine produced the same kind of feverish symptoms on him when he was well as were experienced by people who had malaria. A possible explanation suggested itself: that what had been regarded as the symptoms of disease might in fact be the symptoms of the body's resistance *to* the disease. If so, the aim of treatment should be to assist the symptoms homeopathically, rather than try to suppress them allopathically; lending credibility to the age-old idea of likes curing likes.

It was not, admittedly, the same idea which had often been put forward and acted upon in the past: that a plant which had a flower in the shape of an ear should be used to treat earache. But Hahnemann's version had in fact been presented before, from time to time; in the Hippocratic writings, and in Sydenham's treatise. However unpleasant symptoms might appear, Sydenham had observed, they could be nature's way of trying to 'throw off the morbific matter, and thus recover the patient'. He had not, though, made the deduction Hahnemann now made, following experiments on himself, and on any friends who were ready to volunteer, trying out the effects of drugs on them while they were well and noting the symptoms, thereby 'proving' the drugs, and showing that they could be used to treat illnesses with similar symptoms.

An English country doctor, Edward Jenner, happened at the time to be investigating a folk-lore tradition which, when it proved to be valid, provided some confirmation of Hahnemann's thesis. In oriental countries a variety of methods had been used to protect people from severe smallpox by inoculating them with pus taken from a mild variety. Early in the eighteenth century Lady Mary Wortley Montagu, wife of the British Ambassador to Turkey, had her own children inoculated there; and on her return had persuaded the Princess of Wales to have her own children inoculated too. The problem had been that as the inoculation was from person to person other disorders, like syphilis, might be transmitted. Jenner heard a dairymaid claim that she could not get smallpox because she had had cowpox, a mild disorder bringing nothing worse than a slight malaise and a rash. Finding that the evidence from his country practice appeared to confirm the truth of her statement, Jenner decided to experiment by 'vaccinating' a boy with cowpox pus, and then infecting him with smallpox. Fortunately for Jenner, whose medical qualifications were flimsy, the experiment was a success; and he was hailed as a great innovator.

Vaccination was, in a sense, a testimonial to homeopathy; Hahnemann had, in fact, thought of trying a similar experiment but had discarded the idea because he felt that the risks were too great. And the enthusiasm with which Jenner's innovation was greeted suggests that if Hahnemann had been content simply to expound his idea of likes curing likes, though for a time they would have created violent controversy, he too might now be with Jenner in orthodoxy's Pantheon. But he had begun to test the effects of different dosages of drugs; and he found that diluting the strength by succussion – shaking up the drug in water, or in some other solution – seemed to increase rather than diminish a drug's potency. It appeared to be at its most effective, he claimed, when in chemical terms it had virtually ceased to exist. And when in 1810 he published his *Organon of Rational Healing*, it presented the case not just for homeopathic treatment, but also for treatment with diluted, succussed, 'potentised' drugs.

To medical scientists this was crazy. How could diluting a drug potentize it? Obviously it must have the opposite effect! But if Hahnemann's theory took the public's fancy in the way Mesmer's had it would make orthodox polypharmacy, with its blunderbuss compound drugs, look ridiculous, and jeopardise the reputations of doctors who prescribed them. It would also seriously diminish the incomes of the apothecaries. Even Mesmer had not suffered so malignant a storm of abuse in Austria as fell on Hahnemann; and in 1820 a court ruling prohibited him from continuing his practice.

The prosecution was the result of a reconciliation between the Leipzig physicians and apothecaries. Relations between them had long been strained: the physicians felt that an apothecary ought to confine himself to making up the prescriptions which each patient brought to him following a visit to their consulting rooms; the apothecaries felt that they themselves could prescribe more effectively, and at much less cost to the patient, than any physician. Mutual detestation of homeopathy brought them together; and they were encouraged by the news that Francis I of Austria, on the advice of his doctors, had banned the practice of homeopathy within his empire.

Hahnemann was charged with dispensing medicine – instead of, as the law laid down, prescribing it and leaving it to be dispensed by an apothecary. In his defence Hahnemann pointed out that the need for this law had arisen because the compounding of allopathic drugs had become so difficult and skilled a craft; such skill was not needed for homeopathic preparations, and insofar as experience *was* needed, the apothecaries certainly did not have it. The court disagreed. Hahnemann, the verdict was, must cease to dispense his remedies, under penalty of a fine – with more serious consequences to follow if he disobeyed.

By this time, however, Hahnemann had attracted some influential supporters, among them Prince Schwarzenburg, generalissimo of the allied forces which had defeated Napoleon at the battle of Leipzig seven years earlier. Schwarzenburg was still in his forties but ill-health – brought on, it was believed, by his excesses – had plagued him; when conventional bleedings and purgings proved unavailing he had decided to try Hahnemann's treatment; a decision which amused Goethe when he heard about it. 'A curious game is being played by refusing and damming up innovations of every kind,' he commented. 'It is forbidden to cure by magnetism, and nobody is allowed to practise by Hahnemann's method.' As a result Schwarzenburg, 'very ill and probably incurable' had had to beg for leave of absence from the Emperor 'to seek a cure from across the border' – in Leipzig. When the Emperor agreed, the King of Saxony could hardly snub so illustrious a visitor; and he ordered that no further steps should be taken against Hahnemann. Schwarzenburg came to Leipzig; and to the mortification of the local physicians and apothecaries Hahnemann's treatment worked. Its beneficial results were not lasting: feeling better, Schwarzenburg went back not merely to his former self-indulgence but also, when it began to take its toll, to bleedings and purgings; and soon he was dead. An attempt was made to shift the blame for his death on to homeopathy; but it was unavailing. The risk that the law might make it impossible for Hahnemann to continue to practise had narrowly been averted.

From the start Hahnemann had admitted that he could not justify his belief that dilution and succussion potentised drugs on any abstract ground. 'This doctrine,' he reiterated in a reply to his critics written in 1825, 'insists on wanting to be judged from experience.' Six years later the opportunity arose: the great cholera epidemic reached Europe from India. Hahnemann's explanation of how the disease spread was half-a-century in advance of his time. 'The stuffy spaces of ships, filled as they are with musty aqueous vapours,' he surmised, would be the breeding ground 'for an enormously increased swarm of those infinitely small, invisible, living organisms which are so hostile to human life, and which most probably form the matter of cholera.' The remedies he proposed had been devised from basic homeopathic principles even before the first cases of cholera were reported in Austria; and reports quickly suggested that they were decidedly more successful than any form of treatment which orthodoxy offered. Cardinal Veith, a qualified doctor as well as a priest, preached sermons in homeopathy's favour in the cathedral in Vienna; the Imperial ban was openly ignored; and the testimonials it received led to homeopathic theory and practise attracting attention in other European countries, in Britain and in the United States.

ANIMAL MAGNETISM

For a time it appeared that animal magnetism might also confound its orthodox critics. Mesmer had died in 1815, but some of his disciples had continued to use his methods – though with one significant departure from his principles. Convulsions and dissociation, Puységur had found, were not essential in the treatment of illness. Patients could be put into a light trance, similar to the condition of sleep-walking in which people who are asleep behave and act as if awake. In this condition the mesmerised 'somnabulist' became highly suggestible. If told that his symptoms would disappear he would often, when he came out of his trance, exclaim that they *had* disappeared. In particular the 'magnetisers' – or 'mesmerists', as they came to be called in English-speaking countries – found it was a relatively simple matter to relieve or remove pain.

Although the pain-killing effects of nitrous oxide and of ether were known, their potential as anesthetics had not been grasped. Mesmerism consequently offered the only available prospect of pain-free surgery; and when in the 1820's the French Academies were persuaded to undertake another enquiry into animal magnetism, members of the investigating committee were given a demonstration. Although they were hardly less sceptical than their predecessors of the 1780's they saw that a woman who had been 'magnetised' showed no sign of discomfort while a surgical operation was performed to remove a breast tumour, and heard her explain after it that she had felt no pain. They had to concede in their report that there had been no deception; the method worked.

If the mesmerists had been content to demonstrate the method's pain-killing properties, it is just possible that orthodoxy might grudgingly have accepted it for this purpose, enabling it to be eased gradually into clinical respectability. But they had found further possible uses. While in their trance states some somnambulist subjects seemed to acquire second sight; and one girl who had the faculty of becoming clairvoyant in this way demonstrated to the investigators from the Academies that although she had no medical training she could diagnose what was the matter with certain patients better than medically-qualified physicians had been able to do. This proved to be too much for the Academies, when the investigators reported. It smacked of a revival of the occultism which they thought had finally been demolished by science. The report was repudiated; another committee was set up whose members could be relied upon to reverse its findings; and after a cursory survey of the evidence, they did.

So although fifteen years were to go by before anesthetics came into general use in surgery, the alternative offered by the mesmeric trance state was everywhere ignored by the medical profession. From time to time individual surgeons were persuaded to try it; but whenever its advantages were demonstrated they were attributed to collusion between the patient and the mesmerist. Mesmerism, the fashionable London surgeon Sir Benjamin Brodie explained, was no more than 'a debasing superstition', the real explanation being that almost anyone could 'sustain bodily suffering without any outward expression of what he suffers', and a similar explanation was given by the celebrated physiologist Marshall Hall to the Royal Medical and Chirurgical Society, following a demonstration in 1842.

The patient had had a leg amputated without moving a muscle; if he had been genuinely unconscious, Hall explained, his other leg would have twitched in sympathy during the operation. Later, Hall told the society that his suspicions had been confirmed; he had heard that the patient had confessed to being a party to the deception. The patient wrote indignantly to deny that he had made any such confession; he would like to testify that he had felt no pain. Hall told the Society that as he had heard about the confession from 'the most honourable and truthful of men', who had himself heard about it from 'a person in whom he had full confidence', he felt that the Society should accept his word for it, rather than the patient's. The members agreed, refusing to hear the patient's testimony; a verdict which the *Lancet* praised as 'impartial'.

How could otherwise honourable and reasonable men come to behave in this way? There was one excuse for them. Mesmer's disciples had continued to believe in animal magnetism, the magnetic 'fluid' which, they assumed, came from space and could be transmitted through the mesmerist to the patient. And they also believed, as Mesmer had, that objects could be 'magnetised', and keep that property – much as a magnetised iron bar would keep it. In the United States in the 1790's Elisha Perkins had introduced metallic tractors – rods which could be used for this purpose; and his son brought them over to Britain, where they commanded a high price. A Bath doctor, John Haygarth, decided to test them by substituting unmagnetised tractors, exactly resembling Perkins' without telling anybody. When the bogus tractors were applied four out of five patients said they felt much relieved; which was taken to be clear confirmation of the earlier verdict of the French Academicians, that such cures were the product of the imagination.

Forty years later John Elliotson was caught out in much the same way. Whereas Perkins might simply have been a clever entrepreneur, though, there could be no question in Elliotson's case of deliberate deception. He was greatly admired both as an innovator – he had introduced Laennec's stethoscope to Britain, and helped to found University College Hospital – and as a physician. Originally sceptical about mesmerism, Elliotson had been convinced of its value by demonstrations, and began to demonstrate it himself with the help of a piece of nickel, a metal which he thought was particularly magnetisable. As a test Thomas Wakley, the editor of the *Lancet*, substituted a piece of unmagnetised nickel. When the subject went into a trance, he denounced her as a cheat who was only pretending to be mesmerised; the implication being that Elliotson must be either himself a cheat, or a dupe.

For Elliotson the setback was only temporary. Instructed by the University College Hospital authorities to stop using mesmerism he preferred to resign; but he could continue to practise as a doctor, looking after – among others – Dickens and Thackeray, both of whom revered him. He had had enough experience of mesmerism to know that trickery could not be the explanation; and in the magazine that he founded, the *Zoist*, he continued to record evidence of its effectiveness. But orthodox physicians assumed that mesmerism had been finally discredited. It did not matter how often it was demonstrated; the results were either ignored, or dismissed as obtained by fraud.

WATER CURE

It was possible for orthodox physicians to rationalise their fear and hatred of Mesmer and Hahnemann by claiming that what they practised, being derived from fallacious theories, must be harmful. Another innovator in the early part of the nineteenth century was less easy to dispose of on this pretext: Vincenz Priessnitz of Grafenburg, in Bohemia

Priessnitz re-established what would now be described as naturopathy, or nature cure; with particular emphasis on cold water, taken internally and externally. Not that 'taking the waters' had ever ceased to be an attraction: Spa, in the Ardennes, had become fashionable following a visit in 1717 by Peter the Great of Russia (a plaque recorded that he had been restored to health 'having happily drunk of these most healthful springs'). Bath, too, became fashionable again in the course of the eighteenth century. Watering places of this kind, though, were really resorts, which the well-to-do could attend with the agreeable excuse that they were not really on holiday, because they were doing what their doctors had ordered. They could also be attended by a doctor while they were there. The regimen at Priessnitz's establishment was more spartan; and he had neither medical qualifications nor medically qualified assistants.

Priessnitz believed that water had healing power. Patients were sponged down with cold mountain water, wrapped in wet sheets, plunged into icy baths or sluiced down with douches falling from many feet above to ensure maximum impact. Patients were also expected to drink the water in large quantities, and to take plenty of fresh air and exercise. To judge from surviving comments little care was taken with diet; the food was described by one British visitor as 'the usual alternations of the greasy and the sour met with at German tables'. And the living quarters were squalid. But in other respects it was the forerunner of today's nature cure establishments, notably in the prohibition of any drugs or stimulants, even coffee.

The Austrian physicians refused to believe that Priessnitz was telling the truth when he said that nothing but pure mountain water was used in his treatments. Four times in the 1820's he was taken to court on charges that he was practising medicine while unqualified; but the contents of sponges which had been smuggled in to collect the evidence from his establishment showed no signs of being tampered with or polluted in any way, and the health record of his patients, even during epidemics, was good enough to make it impossible to trap him on that account. Three times he was acquitted; and although following the fourth prosecution he was found guilty and sentenced to a term of imprisonment, the verdict was overturned on appeal.

Despairing of the courts, the physicians turned to the Court: the Imperial authorities were persuaded to set up a commission to investigate the water cure. So favourable were its findings that Priessnitz was granted what almost amounted to the same rights as physicians; and the publicity attracted numerous new patients, including members of the Austrian aristocracy, and curious visitors from other parts of Europe.

Chapter Three

THE CLOSED SHOP

Priessnitz, however, was an embarrassment rather than a threat to the medical Establishment. Homeopathy was a different matter; and wherever it spread it was treated by orthodox physicians as if it were itself a plague. Hahnemann died in 1843, but the campaigns of denigration and vilification continued, the success of his method in the first cholera epidemic being attributed to rumours disseminated by his disciples. In 1854, however, cholera again spread through Europe; and the fact that a homeopathic hospital had been opened in London made it possible to compare its results in treating the disease (its wards were given over to cholera cases) with those of other London hospitals, because the newly-founded Board of Health sent inspectors round all of them. The inspector assigned to the Homeopathic Hospital was compelled to admit that the treatment worked; 'Although an allopath in principle, education and practice,' he wrote, 'were it the will of Providence to afflict me with cholera and deprive me of the power of prescribing for myself, I would rather be in the hands of a homeopathic than an allopathic adviser.'

This was not calculated to please his colleagues on the Board, and when the statistics which had been collected during the epidemic were conveyed to Parliament they omitted the relevant figures from the Homeopathic Hospital. A young member of Parliament, Lord Grosvenor, spotted the deficiency, and the Board was ordered to furnish all the returns which it had collected. They showed that the average mortality among cholera patients had been over fifty per cent – except in the Homeopathic Hospital, where it had been sixteen point four per cent. Called upon to explain why they had suppressed this information, the members of the committee explained they had unanimously decided that if the statistics were made public, 'They would give an unjustified sanction to an empirical practice alike opposed to the maintenance of truth and to the progress of science.'

HYPNOTISM

That the medical Establishment should have felt compelled to try to rig the evidence in this fashion was the measure of its fear, at the time, that the foundations of rational truth and science were being undermined by a revival of occultism. For a while in the 1840's it had seemed possible that the threat had been removed; but this had proved to be an illusion.

In 1843 a book was published with the odd title *Neurypnology*, its author – a hard-headed Scots surgeon, James Braid – arguing that the mesmeric trance state was genuine, and that it could be put to good therapeutic purposes by the medical profession. No matter how convincing the evidence, a book with such a theme and title would ordinarily have stood little chance of carrying conviction; but Braid provided a more plausible theory about how mesmerism worked. It was not, he insisted, animal magnetism or any other occult force that put subjects into a trance. The trance could be induced simply by getting them to gaze at, say, a bright object. This, he suggested, triggered off a neurological response in the brain, which in turn was responsible for the convulsions, and the other phenomena. (It also incidentally explained the reactions to Elliotson's nickel. When subjects had once been hypnotised, Braid had found, it might not be necessary to go through the whole procedure again to put them into a trance: a word, or a gesture – or by extension, the sight of the mesmerist holding out the familiar piece of nickel – might set them off.)

Rationalists, therefore, at last had an excuse to accept mesmerism, purged of its former associations. But there was one snag: Braid had also found a few patients who responded to his gestures even if they could not see what he was doing, in the way Jussieu had observed sixty years earlier. They could even describe objects held behind their backs. As the last thing Braid wanted was to wreck the prospects of his idea finding acceptance by having to admit it was still tainted with occultism, he offered the ingenious explanation that under hypnosis (as he decided to call the mesmeric trance) some people enjoyed greatly heightened perception, so that they could *feel* what was behind them, even if they could not see it.

Braid's idea was taken up by W. B. Carpenter, Professor of Physiology at London University, author of what was becoming a standard textbook of physiology, and a tireless propagandist for mechanist ideas. If it were impossible to discredit animal magnetism, Carpenter decided, the next best thing was to take it over, and show that the hitherto unexplained phenomena could all be accounted for in terms of hyperacuity of the senses and hyperactivity of the muscles. The mesmeric trance, he agreed, was a neurological phenomenon. In it people were able to make so much more effective use of their five senses that they gave the illusion of having a sixth sense; and also to make so much better use of their muscles that they appeared, like madmen, to have the strength of ten. There was nothing occult about it.

A similar theory was proposed in the United States, soon afterwards; John Bovee Dods attributed the trance to 'electrobiology', suggesting that people who had been 'biologised' – a term which was to enjoy a limited colloquial currency for the next half-century – were, in some fashion, electrified, and it was this that stimulated their faculties. And if further proof were required that mesmerism (whatever the explanation) had a therapeutic role, it was provided by the work of James Esdaile – like Braid, a Scots surgeon. In 1845 he began to employ a mesmerist to help him when he had to carry out operations on the employees of the East India Company in Calcutta; soon he had performed scores of them, painlessly; and a committee of hostile colleagues who investigated the method had to admit in their report that it worked.

Hypnotism, or electro-biology, appeared at last to have a passport to respectability. But it was as if the Fates were determined to intervene. In Boston in 1846 William Morton showed that ether could be successfully employed as an anesthetic in surgery; and when Robert Lister performed the first operation with an anesthetic in Britain his comment, 'this Yankee dodge beats mesmerism hollow', reflected the relief which surgeons felt that they would not, after all, have to learn a technique they had resisted so long, and so vehemently. Soon, too, there was ground for uneasiness about the explanations Braid, Carpenter and Dods had provided, when table-turning became a popular craze, first in the United States and then, in the early 1850's, in Europe. Many of the phenomena had been reported from time to time in connection with mesmerism; but the manifestations associated with Spiritualism were even more striking, and much less easy to rationalise, particularly the way the tables responded to the touch of finger-tips with raps, jerks, shudders, twists, slithering movements and levitations.

So many distinguished citizens, including royalty, were involved that the obvious explanation, trickery, could not suffice. Instead Faraday offered a variant of Carpenter's theory, 'quasi-involuntary muscular action'. As it was hopelessly inadequate to account for what fingertip pressure could do to heavy dining-room tables, and did not even begin to explain why they were often reported as moving when they were not being touched, it was an unconvincing theory; but scientists proceeded to react as they had done before (and would often do again). They declined to investigate the subject further; Faraday, they could claim, had settled the issue. If pressed by anybody who considered that it had not been settled, they attributed whatever could not be explained by quasi-involuntary muscular action to trickery.

The same applied to hypnotism. Medical journals no longer dismissed it out of hand; they simply kept it at arm's length, as a neuro-physiological curiosity of dubious ancestry. A few individuals continued to experiment with it, and a few showmen took the opportunity to tour the halls, hypnotising volunteers and putting them through comic routines to make audiences laugh; but it remained unacceptable as a therapeutic technique.

THE 1858 ACT

In the circumstances, physicians (or 'allopaths', as they were by this time describing themselves) felt justified in rejecting, and wherever possible suppressing, all evidence which conflicted with their assumptions. It would be better, though – they had come to realize – if they had the power to prevent such damaging evidence from being collected; and soon they were offered that power, in a Bill designed to weld British doctors into a united profession with self-regulatory powers of the kind lawyers enjoyed.

Legislation to set up the medical profession had long been urged, and proposals were debated on a number of occasions in Parliament in the mid-1850's. There was general agreement that the whole structure of medical education and organisation needed a drastic overhaul to remove anomalies and injustices. More than twenty licensing bodies were in existence around the country; and this had given the Royal College of Physicians the excuse to cling to its monopoly in and around London on the pretext that some doctors had qualified in medical schools where the standards were too low – the excuse being handy to exclude even the most renowned provincial physicians, whose skill would threaten Londoners' practices.

The Government's aim was to bring some order into what was generally admitted to be chaos. All qualified doctors, whether physicians, surgeons or apothecaries, were to be enrolled on a single Register, with reciprocity of rights to practise between the regions. In order to ensure that it was efficiently compiled and maintained, a General Medical Council would be set up with instructions to make whatever regulations were required to ensure that only suitably qualified individuals would appear in the Register. These proposals sounded so reasonable that they created little stir at Westminster. Only one voice was raised in the Commons to warn of the dangers of giving the medical profession such monopoly powers; and in reply, it could be argued that the Bill was not being pushed through at the behest of doctors, as the Royal College of Physicians was actually opposed to it.

The College's opposition was not in fact based on any

objection to the principle of the Bill. Its members were annoyed that they were being shorn of their privileges; and they resented the fact that physicians would henceforth be bracketed with surgeons and, worse, apothecaries, many of whom had had little or no formal training in medicine. The surgeons did not much care for the enforced marriage with the physicians, either; but they were not prepared to oppose the Bill on that account, contenting themselves with deciding to preserve their identity by retaining the designation 'Mr'. Most of them, probably, shared the physicians' resentment at having to let apothecaries into the profession. But members of parliament had country seats, and needed doctors to look after their families and their retainers. The apothecaries consequently had a powerful lobby. Besides, the physicians and surgeons knew that when the Act came into force there would be little need to worry. The new General Medical Council, which they dominated, could lay down the qualifications; and this would mean they could control entry into the profession.

The Bill went through the Commons without difficulty; but by this time Lord Grosvenor had succeeded to his father's title and, as Lord Ebury, he had a seat in the Lords. In the form it was drafted, he pointed out, it would enable the General Medical Council to disqualify any doctor for using unorthodox methods of treatment; and as this could easily be employed against doctors who chose to practise homeopathy he persuaded the Lords to accept an amendment striking out the clause. Any hope the physicians had of having it reinstated in the Commons was dashed when the Home Secretary admitted that an attempt had already been made, in a Scots medical school, to prevent intending homeopathic doctors from qualifying. A candidate had been told that if he wished to receive a degree he must pledge himself 'utterly and solemnly to renounce the practice of homeopathy'; a promise he had courageously declined to make.

The omission of the clause meant, in effect, that as soon as a student had qualified in Britain he was free to use any form of treatment he liked, provided it kept within the law of the land and did not infringe the profession's ethical code, enforced by the General Medical Council. But this produced less flexibility than might have been expected. Training remained in the hands of the medical schools at Universities and of the teaching hospitals; and they saw to it that a rigid orthodoxy was maintained. To become a homeopathic doctor it was necessary first to qualify as a doctor in the ordinary way, the training being basically allopathic; and in the course of it the student would be unlikely to hear anything about homeopathy except abuse. And although the Act did not attempt to restrict the right of individuals who had no medical qualifications from continuing to practise – unlike some European countries, and some States of the American Union, where the right to treat patients was restricted by law to the medical profession – the General Medical Council could exercise some control over unqualified practitioners by laying down that it would be unethical for a doctor to permit his patients to be treated by anybody who was not on the Register, or a recognised auxiliary. It consequently became more difficult for unqualified practitioners to make a living; most of them had to become part-timers.

Similar laws, often well-intentioned, began to strengthen orthodoxy's control all over the world; and it happened that orthodoxy in this period was becoming more allopathic, and more materialistic, in its assumptions – and also more reductionist. In 1760 Morgagni had shown how it was possible to trace symptoms to faults in specific organs within the body. Forty years later Bichat had made the point that it was not diseased organs which were responsible for the symptoms, but diseased tissues within the organs. And in the 1850's Virchow demonstrated that it was specific cells within the tissues, rather than the tissues, which were the disease carriers. At the same time Claude Bernard was perfecting his theory of the *milieu intérieur*: the body's self-regulatory system, or homeostat, automatically adjusting, stabilising and reconciling the body's operations with the help of hormone messengers, on the same principle that a thermostat operates to maintain a steady temperature. The allopaths could consequently claim that these and other discoveries were demonstrating the essential rightness of their case. Illness must be the consequence of a breakdown in the homeostat, occasioned by disease agents – even if the agents' identity remained unknown.

Advances in scientific knowledge about disease, however, had not led to any substantial improvement in methods of treatment. In surgery the introduction of anesthetics, though sparing patients pain, did nothing to reduce the high mortality rate from infections. Semmelweiss had made the momentous discovery that puerperal fever, with its high death rate, could be virtually eliminated if doctors washed their hands before they examined each patient; but his only reward had been the derision, and worse, of his colleagues, resentful at the implication that they were their patients' executioners.

The great majority of drugs prescribed, too, were still either useless or harmful. Except for wine, opium and a few specifics which doctors could not claim to have discovered, Oliver Wendell Holmes – Professor of Anatomy at Harvard, author and wit – observed in 1860, 'I firmly believe that if the whole *materia medica*, as now used, could be sunk to the bottom of the sea, it would be all the better for mankind – and all the worse for the fishes'; and a few months later the bankruptcy of orthodox treatment was sourly confirmed in the *Times* report of the last hours of Cavour. Three doctors had attended him, between them diagnosing that he was suffering from congestion of the brain, brain fever, typhus, dropsy and the gout; and 'for all these diseases they could think of nothing but their own sovereign remedy – the lancet'. Cavour was bled, and when he got worse, bled again and again, until the only way in which more blood could be taken from him was by compression. 'There never was a clearer case,' the *Times* correspondent lamented, 'of a man murdered by his medical attendants.'

The allopaths' inability to offer more effective and safer methods of treatment kept the vitalists' hopes alive; but they lacked a new, more rational-sounding model to present as an alternative to orthodoxy. Nature cure hardly sufficed, though it retained its popularity. After Priessnitz's death in 1851 his establishment for a time went into a decline; but the regime introduced by the Dominican Father Kneipp, almoner of an Austrian convent, attracted an even more enthusiastic following. Kneipp's prescription was much the same as Priessnitz's, but with the addition of walking barefoot through cold water or, where available, early morning dew or snow – a treatment still recommended in many spas in Europe. In England, Dr Gully's water cure at Malvern became fashionable. Gully courageously tried to combine it with other forms of unorthodox treatment – to Darwin's disgust; greatly though he felt he had benefitted when he took the cure he complained that his 'beloved Dr Gully', when one of his patients was very ill, in addition to his own services as a 'hydropathist', employed 'a clairvoyant girl to report on internal changes, a mesmerist to put her to sleep, and a homeopathist'. Darwin had to admit, though, that the girl had recovered.

Nature cure, however, had never been any great threat to orthodoxy; and homeopathy was ceasing to be, at least in Britain. The protection the homeopaths had been given by the 1852 Act was already proving to be their undoing, because the price they had to pay for remaining members of the medical club had turned out to be exorbitant. Prospective homeopathic practitioners could not be denied entry into the medical profession; but they had to qualify by passing the standard examinations in what was largely allopathic medicine, and in the process they were subjected to a powerful indoctrination against homeopathic teachings. They then had to undertake the further course of training to qualify as homeopathic practitioners; and they might not be able to afford to wait so long before beginning to earn an income. As there were few homeopathic hospitals there was also less incentive to live on a pittance while young in the hope of wealth to come as a consultant later.

Homeopathy was also set back when surgery began to become relatively trouble-free. The introduction of antisepsis in the 1860's led to a massive increase in the number and range of operations, and the replacement of the physician by the surgeon, at least in the patient's eyes, as the leading figure in the medical hierarchy. Homeopathic remedies had traditionally been regarded as rendering surgery unnecessary; and although homeopaths had no prejudice against surgery as such, they made little use of it. To add to their problems they were split by a dispute over potencies. On 'likes cure likes', there was no disagreement. Potencies were a different matter; some homeopaths felt that dilutions and succussion were not always necessary. To purists this was a betrayal; and the wrangle which followed was gleefully exploited by allopaths.

In the United States, where homeopathy was dominated by the influence of James Tyler Kent, this was less of a problem, as he managed to persuade most of his followers to obey Hahnemann's law. He was assisted by the fact that the American Medical Association was not compelled, as the British profession had been, to tolerate homeopathy's existence. The American Medical Association had originally been founded in the 1840's to fight homeopathy; and it continued to do so with unabated rancour until the end of the century, forbidding its members to prescribe homeopathic remedies or to have any dealings with homeopaths. Nevertheless homeopathy continued to flourish; by the turn of the century it was estimated that there were nearly ten thousand practitoners. In 1930 the AMA suddenly relented: homeopaths were invited to join. Feeling that this represented a remarkable victory, as historically it did, they gratefully accepted. From that day on, homeopathy in the United States began to decline.

LOURDES

The Churches, too, elected to try to come to terms with the medical profession rather than fight for the recognition of the clergy as healers. From time to time an individual priest might become a local celebrity, and occasionally more than that: in the mid-nineteenth century the reputation of the Curé d'Ars for miraculous cures led to this village being besieged by pilgrims from all over Europe. But the Vatican continued to abide by the rules laid down by Lambertini; and although it was not formally specified this ordinarily meant that no cure was acceptable as divinely miraculous unless it appeared to have been performed through the intervention of Jesus, Mary, a martyr or a saint, actual or prospective.

Shortly before the Curé d'Ars died in 1859, Bernadette Soubirous had her vision of the Virgin Mary at Lourdes; and

Lourdes soon became the chief magnet for Catholics looking for miraculous cures. How little the Church welcomed the development could be gauged by the severity with which it treated Bernadette; but when it became clear that she would be submissive, leaving all the credit to Mary, a system of control was introduced which was nicely calculated to offend neither the gullible faithful nor those Catholics, increasingly influential, who were sceptical about miracles. The faithful could arrive, singly or in batches, to go through the prescribed rituals and, if they were cured of their diseases, to go home and boast about it to their friends. But no cure would be accepted as divinely miraculous by the Church unless it had been carefully investigated by a committee of doctors convened for the purpose. Only if the committee accepted the evidence might the Vatican, at some later date, give its approval.

As all the records in cases which were investigated were open to inspection the doctors concerned could not easily be accused of approving spurious miracles at the Vatican's behest; and stricter interpretation of Lambertini's guidelines was to mean in practice that many cures which formerly would have been considered miraculous were rejected. The number accepted became so small – one every two years – that it represented little threat to the peace of mind of Catholic doctors, anxious to show that they were as scientifically-minded as their colleagues.

CHRISTIAN SCIENCE

Vitalism, though, was not quite moribund; and in the 1860's it began again to show signs of life in the United States. Mesmerism, old-style, had made little impression there before it had been overtaken by 'electro-biology'; but a few 'magnetisers' used Mesmer's and Puysegur's techniques. One of them, Phineas Quimby of Maine, decided that as he was able to treat patients successfully by this method they ought to be able to treat themselves without the need of a hypnotist to put them into a trance; an idea which attracted Mary Patterson, a chronic invalid, who came to him for treatment in

1862. Even before she had met him, she had written ', disease is in the mind', adding the deduction that 'as disease is what follows the error, destroy the cause and the effect will cease'; but she had not found a way to destroy the cause. Quimby provided it. Cured, she went on after his death to develop her theory, presenting it in 1875 in *Science and Health*. Disease, she contended, is an illusion. It can only exist if an individual believes that it exists: 'If you fill your mind with thoughts of self-confidence, courage, outward activity and interest in the glowing and vital things of life, the morbid ideas will be turned out of doors and there will be no vacant spot to which they can return.' There was consequently no need for doctors, or even for a healer. It might be desirable to have somebody to consult, as she had consulted Quimby. But each individual should aim to render any form of treatment unnecessary by banishing the notion of illness. And in 1879 she set up the first Christian Science Church in Boston, to encourage disciples and to win converts to her faith.

Mary Baker Eddy, as she had become following a further marriage, was even on the most charitable interpretation a domineering and neurotic woman. She could not tolerate rivals, even after they were dead; in her anxiety to show that her ideas were her own, rather than Quimby's, she began to disparage his work, and to equate mesmerism with witchcraft – 'malicious animal magnetism' which, she claimed, was being used against her. But her Church began to flourish, spreading out all over the world. And in retrospect, considering the alternatives – orthodoxy's useless drugs and dangerous bleedings and purgings – the recruits can hardly be considered foolhardy for deciding to join the new cult.

THE MANIPULATORS

Nevertheless it was a cult; and as such an irritation rather than a danger to the medical Establishment. Doctors were more concerned, in this period, by a rival form of therapy designed to supplant standard allopathic methods, and replace them with spinal manipulation.

wagon era in the nineteenth century, when America were being wrested from the Red and converted into white ranches and settlements, ified doctors were few. Primitive training schools came into being to turn out what might be described as hobnailed-boot doctors – apothecaries, vets, bonesetters. One of them, Andrew Taylor Still, went on to pick up experience as an army doctor on the Union side in the Civil War before settling down to practise in the Mid-West. What he had seen of ortho-dox medicine did not impress him; and when three of his own children died in a meningitis epidemic he decided that there must be other, more effective, methods of treatment.

By Still's own account the importance of the spine in treat-ing illness had first been impressed on him when, as a ten-year-old boy, he had got rid of a headache by lying down with his neck on a blanket slung between two trees. If the spine were freed to perform its function of acting as a channel for the nerves, he decided, leaving the nerves free to perform their function of regulating the blood supply through the arteries and veins, nature's healing force would cope with diseases more effectively than any medicine. He began to practise, and later teach, manipulation of the spine to assist the vertebrae to return to their natural alignment; an ex-tension of what bonesetters had traditionally done with speci-fic joints to restore limbs to normal use.

'Osteopathy', as Still called his technique, might conceiv-ably have developed into a recognized therapy in the way dentistry was doing, if he and his disciples had limited them-selves to manipulation for disorders of the spine. But they refused to accept any such limitation, believing that manipula-tion was an effective treatment of disorders of all kinds. To orthodoxy, the idea that jerking or twisting the spinal verte-brae could counter the effects of, say, influenza or indigestion, let alone of TB, seemed insane; and the American Medical Association embarked on an unrelenting campaign to destroy osteopathy by ridicule and, failing that, by legal action. Geo-graphy, however, was against the AMA. In states where there were few doctors, the public came to rely on osteo-paths and to back them when they were persecuted.

Much the same course was taken by chiropractic, an alternative form of spinal manipulation offered a few years later by a 'magnetiser' in the Mesmer tradition, D. D. Palmer. He and his disciples used a different manipulative technique, short sharp thrusts rather than leverage; but they believed in the same fundamental principle that restoring the integrity of the spine would release nature's healing force. As osteopaths graduated to respectability, founding medical schools whose training began to compare favourably with orthodoxy's, chiropractic tended to take over on the hob-nailed boot level, thereby often exciting the same irritation among osteopaths as osteopathy did among doctors. But by the turn of the century both were established in many States, and both were attracting interested observers from European countries, some of whom elected to stay on and undertake the training before going home to practise.

Unscientific though the theory sounded, and can still be made to sound, spinal manipulation was less likely to do harm than many of the orthodox treatments of the time. It will never be known how many people who were assumed to have died of disease were in fact orthodoxy's victims; but as Mark Twain suggested in *Pudd'nhead Wilson*, cradles must have often been emptied because of what the doctor, 'with his antediluvian methods', prescribed.

CHARCOT

Several years were to go by before osteopathy and chiropractic made any impression across the Atlantic; but in Europe in the 1880's the medical Establishment had to face a revival of mesmerism, in the form of hypnotism or 'Braidism', as it was commonly called by its practitioners on the Continent, to distinguish it from 'animal magnetism', still the colloquial usage. And of all the twists and turns in the history of medicine, the rise and fall of hypnotism as a therapy is one of the strangest.

In spite of the backing of Carpenter, Braid's theory of hypnosis had failed to win acceptance in Britain. But it had attracted more attention in France where a few doctors had began to use it, including A. A. Liébeault, modestly practising near Nancy. Liébeault offered to treat patients free if they would let him hypnotise them; and as most of them were peasants, who knew how expensive drugs were, he had no shortage of volunteers. He put them into a light trance, and suggested that their symptoms – headaches, indigestion, or what they might be suffering from – would clear up, which they did often enough for his fame to begin to spread.

Although Liébeault's attempt to publicise his method by writing a book on the subject was a failure, some doctors working at the Salpêtrière Hospital in Paris became interested in the 1870s, among them Jean-Martin Charcot. A neurologist, Charcot experimented with hypnotism to study the interaction of physical and psychological forces; and what he saw convinced him not merely that the hypnotic trance state was genuine (which orthodoxy still denied) but that it might be of great value in finding out precisely how the mind affects the body in sickness and in health.

That emotional crises could precipitate illness had not, up to that time, been seriously questioned. 'My life,' the eighteenth century surgeon John Hunter had remarked, 'is at the mercy of any fool who shall put me in a passion' – an accurate forecast, as he died at an exasperating Board Meeting. The cantankerous Benjamin Rush, Physician-General to Washington's forces and one of the signatories of the Declaration of Independence, admitted that he was fascinated by the way in which disorders could be almost miraculously cleared up by the arousal of some strong emotion, such as fear; he could not account for it, but 'to see the whole system in a moment, as it were, undergo a perfect and entire change, and the most inveterate and incurable disease radically expelled, is surely a very singular and marvellous event'. He had seen many people 'of infirm and delicate habits', too, 'restored to perfect health by the change of place or occupation to which the war exposed them'.

In view of the known ways in which the emotions could cause physical symptoms – nervousness producing a desire to urinate, embarrassment causing a blush, alarm sending up the pulse rate – it had seemed reasonable to speculate that excess of emotion might be a cause of illness. In cases of tuberculosis it was taken for granted: writing to Fanny Brawne, Keats claimed that even if he had any chance of recovery his passion for her would kill him. The publication in 1860 of a pioneering work on 'psychophysics' by the German philosopher-physicist Fechner opened up the prospect of a more scientific study of the whole subject; and Daniel Hack Tuke's *Illustrations of the Influence of the mind upon the body in health and disease*, published twelve years later, carried this development a stage further, containing as it did a section on what he termed 'psycho-therapeutics,' illustrating various ways, including hypnotism, by which the power of the mind could be invoked to assist in the treatment of physical diseases.

Tuke and Charcot were friends; and Charcot had decided to see what would happen if he used hypnosis on hysteric patients. Of all disorders, hysteria was the one which at the time was causing the medical profession most concern. Not that it was lethal, like TB or cholera; but it was a standing reproach to doctors, because it appeared to mock them, manifesting itself as it did in such diverse forms ('the Protean disease', in Sydenham's view). One of the commonest was loss of control over the muscles, leading either to convulsions or paralysis. What would now be regarded as neuroses, presonality disorders of all kinds other than actual mental derangement, were also classified as hysteria. But neurologists were chiefly worried by the remarkable ability of hysterics to mimic the symptoms of other disorders so perfectly that it was often impossible to be sure that they were not suffering from the real thing.

As Freud was to recall in his obituary of Charcot, the nuisance value of hysteria had brought it into discredit, relating not only to the patients but to 'the physicians who treated this neurosis'. It was courageous of Charcot to undertake research into the subject at all, let alone to employ hypnotism, which was still under the Academy's formal interdict. He managed, however, to combine convincing demonstrations that hypnotism was genuine with equally convincing demonstrations of the process by which hysterics produced their symptoms. Having first carefully established which patients really were hysterics by introducing tests of a kind which the medical profession had previously lacked, he was able to show that through suggestion under hypnosis they could be made to mimic the symptoms of other disorders.

When, in 1883, a vacancy occurred in the Academy Charcot presented his thesis so shrewdly that he was elected. Hypnotism, it could be claimed, was now at long last accepted. But to win acceptance for it Charcot had paid a price. The hypnotic state, his research showed, was itself a form of hysteria : a neurological disorder. The convulsions which often accompanied it were due to hysterical 'neuro-muscular hyper-excitability'; and the trance itself was 'induced hystero-epilepsy'. Small wonder, then, that the Academicians had been won over. Annoying though it might be that hypnosis had been shown to be genuine, Charcot had also reassured them that it was of no therapeutic significance; for who would want to induce hystero-epilepsy?

Hardly had Charcot's proposition won acceptance, though, than it was challenged by Professor Bernheim of Nancy. Hearing that Liébeault was treating patients successfully with hypnotism, Bernheim had paid him a visit. Bernheim had expected to be able to expose a charlatan; in the event he had been converted by what he witnessed, and had begun to use hypnotism himself in his Nancy hospital. Liébeault had treated thousands of patients by simple suggestion under hypnosis, and the Nancy hospital was now treating many more : was Charcot seriously suggesting that they were all hysterics? Obviously the fact he had been working exclusively with hysterics had misled him.

Soon even Charcot's dedicated Salpêtrière disciples were forced to admit that Bernheim was right. Once again the way seemed open for mesmerism, in the form that Puységur had pioneered and Liébeault had perfected, to win acceptance. But again the Fates intervened. Liébeault had believed that there was nothing occult about the healing process, a point which Bernheim had been careful to emphasise. But in the course of some experiments, Liébeault and some colleagues found that they could hypnotise patients without the patients being aware of it. This was not new: it had often been reported by the early mesmerists, who had attributed it to thought-transference. But thought-transference – or telepathy, as it was now renamed – was anathema. When it was reported by a doctor treating a patient with hysteria in Le Havre, the young Pierre Janet went down to investigate, expecting to find some explanation which would fit Charcot's theory. Instead, he found that not merely could she react when the hypnotist was in another room – he might be in another house, half-a-mile away, and she would still react as if she was receiving his instructions.

If the practitioners of hypnotism had been able to rally behind Bernheim, using the technique in the treatment of illness and repudiating any link with occultism, it would have stood a better chance of winning general acceptance. But the mass of evidence which appeared in the 1880s, confirming that hypnotism in some unexplained fashion appeared to liberate psychic forces, telepathy and clairvoyance, only succeeded in making it once again suspect. And as it was no longer possible for the medical Establishments in Europe and America to deny that the hypnotic trance state existed they clung to Charcot's explanation, even after he and his Salpêtrière team had been forced to abandon it. To the Establishments, whether his theory was right or wrong mattered little; its value was that it relieved them of any necessity to examine, let alone to employ, hypnotism.

When a committee of enquiry was set up by the British Medical Association to investigate, its members reported to the BMA's annual meeting in 1892 that following visits to Paris and Nancy, they could confirm that hypnotism really was an effective form of treatment. The BMA, shocked, voted that the report should be marked simply 'received'; in other words, it was not 'accepted'. And although individual doctors continued to use hypnotism, and a few researchers, particularly in France, continued to produce evidence of its therapeutic effectiveness, it was ignored by the profession as a whole. 'No-one repudiated hypnotism,' Janet recalled years later. 'No-one denied the power of suggestion'; people simply ceased to talk about them. Or if they did discuss the subject it was in the very different context of the sensation caused by Du Maurier's enormously successful *Trilby*, published in 1895. In the public's mind's eye the hypnotist became a sinister Svengali, with power to sacrifice his unlucky victims to his designs.

The collapse of hypnotism's challenge to orthodoxy was to have far-reaching consequences. It was not simply that members of the medical profession deprived themselves of a potentially useful therapeutic aid. In doing so they took a further step towards accepting that medicine was concerned only with physical, 'organic' illness, over which the mind had no control. Charcot, the belief was, had demonstrated that the mind could induce imitation symptoms; but real symptoms could be caused only by disease agents. And the results of Pasteur's researches had at last provided what the allopaths had been waiting for: proof that disease *was* transmitted by such agents.

Pasteur's discoveries also held out renewed hope of finding better ways to prevent and treat disease. By the 1880s the work of dedicated public servants, Chadwick, Southwood Smith and others, had shown how effective better hygiene and sanitation could be in preventing epidemics; and Koch's isolation of the tubercle bacillus, in 1882, was followed by the discovery of the pathogens of cholera, diptheria, tetanus, pneumonia and meningitis, suggesting that the sources of all infectious disorders would soon be traced. When in 1890 Koch announced the discovery of his tuberculin, designed to provide immunity against TB, it could confidently be expected that successors would follow, and they did. The results, admittedly, were disappointing, and in the case of tuberculin, destructive; but this, time would surely remedy.

For most doctors, therefore, the indications appeared to be that the mind, or the emotions, need no longer be regarded as playing any significant role in disease either as cause or cure. Significantly, when the influential Wilhelm Wundt took on Fechner's 'psycho-physics', he renamed it 'physiological psychology'. Where Fechner, like Charcot, had explored the mind-body relationship, Wundt and his disciples concentrated upon seeking to fit psychology into the mechanistic framework of physiology and physics, which by this time were regarded by medical scientists as allied disciplines. 'Most of the great advances in medical diagnosis in the present day,' Sir William Gardner told the British Medical Association in his Presidential Address in 1888, 'involve applications of pure physics'; in a very few years, he predicted, the physics laboratory 'would become an absolutely essential preliminary step in the education of the physician of the future, and those who have not undergone this training will be hopelessly outdistanced in the race'.

This was far from being Charcot's opinion. In an article he wrote on 'the faith that heals' for the *New Review* just before his death in 1893, he admitted that there were limitations to the power of the mind over the body: 'Faith will never restore an amputated limb.' But not merely could it remove various forms of paralysis; faith could also heal tumours and ulcers, and might be capable of doing still more. Miracles, he urged, should not be dismissed as impossible; they should be studied with a view to understanding how they happened, in case doctors could put the knowledge to good use. It was foolish, he concluded, to imagine 'that at present we know everything in the domain of the supernatural contribution to faith healing'.

Charcot had been listened to with respect so long as he told his audience what they wanted to hear. They did not want to hear that miracles might be attributable to as yet unexplained powers of the mind over the body. They preferred to believe that what he had proved was that the physical symptoms of hysteria or neurosis were 'functional', rather than 'organic'; in other words, the patients were not really ill, or if they were, they were the concern of alienists – the psychiatrists – rather than the neurologist. Only those patients who were too rich or too influential to be told that they were hysterical or neurotic were spared that humiliation. When the eminent lawyer Sir Edward Carson collapsed with one of his periodic bouts of nervous prostration, the diagnosis was neurasthenia: exhausted nerves.

BARKER THE BONESETTER

In Britain, where there was usually a doctor within walking distance and where the medical profession enjoyed a higher social standing than in the United States, there was less opportunity for osteopaths and chiropractors; but individual bonesetters continued to practise. In some areas where there was a large working-class population with few doctors, they flourished. The North of England Friendly Society, of which most miners were members, accepted disability certificates from them on the same basis as from doctors; and a Government enquiry was to testify that though many of them were illiterate they often enjoyed 'a large amount of public confidence'. Occasionally bonesetters would acquire a reputation which would encourage them to move up the financial scale; and in London, a few had acquired fashionable premises and practices.

The 1858 Act did nothing to stop bonesetters from continuing to treat patients; but by laying down that any doctor who sent patients to them could be struck off the Register it converted them from potential allies into rivals, as Sir James Paget realised. In a lecture in 1867 he told students that he proposed to deal with what he called 'the cases that bonesetters cure' – because, he warned, few of them would practise without having a bonesetter as a rival, and 'If he can cure a case which you have failed to cure, his fortune may be made and yours marred.' Paget did not approve of the methods bonesetters commonly used, such as wrenching the joints apart in order to put them back together in their correct alignment. He regarded their theories as misleading, and he feared they did much harm. But he could not dispute that they were often successful. Doctors must learn the techniques for themselves, he insisted, or lose patients; a view which he was to reiterate until his death over thirty years later. But because medical education was hospital-based, students lacked the opportunity to learn bonesetting except where an orthopedic surgeon had troubled to acquaint himself with it, and this was rare.

There was in any case the difficulty that bonesetting could

be an art, up to a point, rather than a craft. And up to a point it could be regarded as vitalist, as the career of the most celebrated of bonesetters, Herbert Barker, was to illustrate. As a youth in the 1880s, on board a liner taking him to Canada, Barker found himself volunteering to 'reduce' – put back in alignment – a passenger's dislocated elbow. He had had no training; it seemed to him that instinct guided him to follow what turned out to be the right procedure. On his return to Britain he apprenticed himself to one of the fashionable London bonesetters, and in due course acquired a fashionable London practice himself. Had he been content to make an affluent living, shunning publicity, he would probably have been left alone; but he boldly challenged the medical profession, persuading the *Daily Express* to sponsor a trial of his methods in which he successfully cured seven out of eight patients whose doctors had said nothing more could be done for them.

The medical Establishment was in no mood, at this time, to allow its authority to be thus challenged. It was stung in 1907 by the production of Shaw's *The Doctor's Dilemma*, with its exposure of quackery within the profession; all the more effective in that, like Molière, Shaw used the formula of black comedy. The General Medical Council could do nothing about Shaw; but the following year it called upon the Government to investigate 'the evil effects produced by the unrestricted practice of medicine and surgery by unqualified persons', and a patient whom Barker had unsuccessfully treated was persuaded to sue him. From the bench, Mr Justice Darling did not attempt to disguise his bias, summing up strongly against Barker; and although the jury awarded the patient derisory damages, the fact that the verdict went against Barker, and that he was ordered to pay the heavy costs, appeared to deal a devastating blow to his reputation and his career.

In all probability both would have been seriously damaged had the General Medical Council not taken the further spiteful step of punishing the doctor who helped him with anesthetics, F. W. Axham, by striking him off the Register. The London newspapers rallied to Barker's side, castigating the GMC, and incidentally giving Barker the publicity which was to revive his spirits and his practice. But the episode showed how perceptive the sole opponent of the 1858 Act in the Commons had been, in warning of the risks of granting the medical profession even a limited monopoly. A valuable form of treatment had been left out of the medical curriculum, yet here was the profession seeking to crush a man for providing it; a man whom even the *Times,* normally to be found on orthodoxy's side, described as having 'effected perfect cures where regular surgeons had failed'.

When Shaw's play was published in book form, reaching a far wider audience than in performance, his preface contained the most virulent attack on the profession's standards that had ever appeared. 'That any sane nation,' he began, 'having observed that you could provide for the supply of bread by giving bakers a pecuniary interest in baking for you, should go on to give a surgeon a pecuniary interest in cutting off your leg, is enough to make one despair of political humanity.' No calculation an astronomer might make about the recurrence of a comet was more certain than that 'under such circumstances we shall be dismembered unnecessarily in all directions by surgeons who believe the operations to be necessary solely because they want to perform them.' Physicians were just as bad, with their superstitious faith in antitoxins, in spite of 'the appalling results which led to the hasty dropping in 1894 of Koch's tuberculin', and other disasters. And not merely did the profession provide a medical service to the community which was 'a murderous absurdity'; it persecuted men of sound sense like Hahnemann and his followers, and foolishly clamoured for the prosecution of Christian Scientists whose dependants had died, forgetting the profession's own death toll.

Barker, though, was the only practitioner who disturbed the peace of mind of the medical profession in Britain in the years before the outbreak of the First World War. Admittedly, as Shaw had observed, the anti-toxins were proving unsatisfactory. Not only had Koch's tuberculin had to be discontinued, the average annual death rate from diphtheria, which had been a hundred and sixty-nine per million persons before its anti-toxin was introduced in 1894, rose to two hundred and seventy-two per million, at a time when the death rate for the other childhood diseases was falling. But there was always the excuse with diphtheria that the death rate would have been even higher without the anti-toxin; and with TB, that a better anti-toxin would soon be found. When in 1911 Ehrlich's 'magic bullet' – Salvarsan – was marketed, it could be hailed as the long awaited break-through. Here was a drug which was specific against syphilis, and effective enough to hold out the promise that chemicals would soon be found which would fulfil Pasteur's expectations that 'all parasitic maladies might be made to disappear from the face of the earth.'

THE GREAT WAR

By the outbreak of the First World War, therefore, the medical profession in Britain and in most of Europe had acquired a large measure of monopoly control; and most unresolved problems could be set aside while attention was concentrated upon preventing outbreaks of disease in the trenches, and dealing with the wounded. Only one minor nuisance remained; a form of hysteria which had long been known as a rarity, but now became disagreeably common in the prolonged trench warfare from 1914 to 1918.

Cases were continually being notified of 'hysterical fugue' – amnesia. The men involved, often experienced and trusted officers or NCOs, would suddenly lose their identity for a few hours, sometimes for weeks or even months. They might wander off from the battlefield, behaving in most respects rationally, and retaining all their faculties except their memory. When they recovered they would have no recollection of what they had been doing in the 'fugue' period. It was clearly hysteria; but by this time the diagnosis of hysteria had become unfashionable. Besides, to have dubbed such men hysterics would have meant having to certify them, and they were not in the ordinary sense insane, even in their fugues. If they were accepted *as* sane, though, they would be subject to court martial, and possibly shot for desertion. A little ingenuity prompted the solution: 'shell-shock'. The bursting of a shell close to the soldier, or the effect of a prolonged bombardment, might have done neurological damage which could be held responsible, enabling the doctors to classify sufferers from fugue as requiring hospital treatment. Once again, a way had been found to keep medicine on its new physiological tramlines.

Chapter Four

BETWEEN THE WARS

The most resounding triumph won by quacks – as they were still commonly regarded and called – in the 1920's, was the vindication of Herbert Barker. During the war he had offered his services to the army: the War Office had refused them, explaining that it was contrary to King's Regulations to employ a medically unqualified practitioner. He had nevertheless treated people in the forces privately, without charging a fee. When, to get around the difficulty, Bernard Shaw suggested that some university might offer Barker an honorary degree in medicine, a spokesman for the General Medical Council replied that if Barker wanted medical qualifications there was nothing to stop him taking a degree in the ordinary way. Shaw was provoked into one of his characteristic explosions. Here, he complained, was 'a surgical manipulator of genius forbidden to treat our disabled soldiers, not because it is denied that he has mastered a valuable technique omitted from the regulation equipment, but simply because the profession is too preoccupied with its own privileges'. To protect itself the profession was relying on an examination system 'which annually lets loose the most disastrous duffers in the sick rooms of the nation'; if the same principle operated in another field 'Brahms and Joachim would have been refused their honorary degrees as doctors of music unless they had stopped composing and playing for five years to pass an Arts examination; do exercises in counterpoint to the satisfaction of professors incapable of writing three bearable bars of original music; and qualify themselves to name, on demand, the age at which Bach's fourth son was christened.'

As no university responded Shaw put forward another proposal: that the Archbishop of Canterbury should use the right, preserved for him under the 1858 Act, to give medical degrees. And after the war ended three hundred past and sitting members of parliament signed a petition urging him to make such an award. Though declining to venture on such a precedent the Archbishop expressed the hope that Barker's 'eminent services' would obtain recognition by some other means; and in 1922, Barker received a knighthood.

Here was the GMC's opportunity to make some amends. His anesthetist, Axham, in his eighties, no longer practised; but it would have been a conciliatory gesture to restore his name to the Register, a course publicly urged by King George V's physician, Lord Dawson of Penn. The GMC refused. Its members could not claim that this was a matter of principle because they had not dared to strike at Axham's successor, knowing as they did that any move in that direction would have led to legislation to curtail their powers, and in all probability radically to change the GMC's composition (a reform that was effectively to be delayed for over half a century). Nevertheless they refused the request, and Axham died a few weeks later.

Yet Barker ought to have been the least of the medical Establishment's worries. He had made no attempt to proselytise, or to set up a training scheme to enable other medically unqualified manipulators to follow his example. On the contrary, he longed for recognition by the profession; and the knighthood appeared to represent a step in that direction, particularly as he knew he had the backing of a few of the most eminent of the physicians and surgeons of the day. It was no help to him because in the long run, his backers could not command a majority on the GMC. Always its members' argument was that though they had nothing against Barker or his techniques, to accord recognition to an unqualified practitioner would be the thin edge of the wedge. If one bonesetter were to be allowed to practise under the protection of some equivalent of the Lambeth degree, others would inevitably follow. Why, even radiesthetists would be seeking admission:

the Abbé Mermet with his absurd pendulum; Albert Abrams with his infamous 'Black Box'!

RADIESTHESIA

Radiesthesia represented a development from practices which in their primitive form were then being reported by investigators of tribal communities all over the world. Basically it was divination: the use of extra-sensory, or unexplained, faculties and powers to diagnose and treat illness. And the various gadgets which were found in use by tribal doctors often resembled those which a few people continued to employ for divination in Europe: pendulums, or crystal balls.

For some reason, however, divination had rarely been heard of in Europe in connection with illness, except at the village crone level. Its most familiar purpose was the location of underground sources of water: 'dowsing', as it was called in Britain. Some dowsers used their bare hands (as some Indian medicine men also did), explaining that they could feel a kind of current passing through them when they were over a source: but most used a pendulum or a forked hazel twig to amplify the 'signal'. Dowsing had often been demonstrated, sometimes with striking success. But it had been suspect because of its occult associations (as the American term for it, 'water-witching', indicated) until in 1854 the French scientist Michel-Ange Chevreul formulated the proposition that the movements of the twig or pendulum were produced not by spirits, but by 'a muscular action which is not the product of will, but the result of a thought carried over to a phenomenon of the outside world' – a parallel hypothesis to the 'unconscious muscular action' suggested by Carpenter to account for table-turning.

Chevreul's theory need not have been regarded as condemnatory of dowsers. On the contrary, insofar as it suggested the possibility that they had found a way to gain access to lost instincts, it might be considered to have disclosed a valuable asset. But it would take time for the prejudice against dowsing to die down; and orthodox scientists were too busy exploring material forces to concern themselves with such unexplained channels of the mind. Paradoxically, though, it was as a consequence of their exploration that dowsing was to be adapted for use in treatment. The discovery of radiations – forces hitherto unknown, but allowing communication at great distances as if by a materialist form of telepathy; and vision through solid objects like human flesh as if by a materialist version of clairvoyance – prompted the idea that radiations would be found which would not merely account for the dowser's ability to find water, but would also enable the method to be applied to diagnose and treat the sick.

By Mermet's own account it occurred to him around 1905, while he was still a parish priest, that as inanimate objects could be detected with the help of a pendulum, it should be possible to apply the same technique to human beings. Veins and arteries could be likened to subterranean streams. Bones, flesh and nerves could be imagined as having certain analogies with various underground 'strata'. The notion set him experimenting, and he found that the pendulum reacted in a different manner when he held it over the body of a sick person from when he held it over somebody who was in good health. Soon he was able to detect the organ which was giving the trouble. Human bodies, he suggested, are constantly emitting radiations which can be detected by means of a current flowing through the hands of the diviner. The pendulum could be used not merely to make the current manifest, but also to facilitate a more accurate diagnosis, because the pendulum 'bob' would swing or rotate consistently, performing in one way for, say, a diseased liver, and another for a diseased spleen.

Because of his vocation, Mermet was able to demonstrate his technique without falling foul of the medical authorities in hospitals; and there were many accounts of the way in which he confounded sceptics. A Liège lawyer described in 1926 how at a cancer hospital in Louvain, Mermet was taken to a ward with ten patients 'completely covered up to the chin, and consequently giving no clue as to the localisation of their tumours': yet in eight of them he had been able to indicate the affected organ; and in the other two, although his diagnosis did not accord with that of the doctors, he was able to argue that the manifestations they had found were secondaries, the primary focus being where he had claimed it to be.

Impressive though his resuts often were, the sight of a priest standing by patients' beds in a hospital ward, holding a pendulum over them, was not calculated to inspire conviction in the minds of most doctors; and when he found a way to avoid the necessity of going to the bedside, though it spared them embarrassment and often humiliation where he was right and they were wrong, it only served to bring his method into greater disrepute. The patient did not have to be present, he claimed, when radiesthesia – the term he introduced for medical dowsing – was being used. Held over a letter written by, or a photograph of, the patient, the pendulum was capable of giving a correct diagnosis. This was an idea he had picked up from 'map dowsers', who believed they could detect the presence of underground water or minerals just as satisfactorily by dowsing over a map of the area as by fieldwork. But doctors who might have been prepared to admit the possibility of an unexplained intuitive force providing some individuals with an affinity for underground water, or for picking up pathological signals from the human body, often jibbed at the notion that such information could be gleaned from a photograph.

The medical Establishment, too, was unhappy at the way in which Mermet and those who took up his method began to apply it in treatment, as well as in diagnosis. Mermet himself insisted that treatment 'must be exclusively reserved for doctors who, after a long course of studies, have acquired the necessary knowledge of the human body and the right of curing diseases' : the trained radiesthesist must always regard himself as a medical auxiliary, never undertaking a case without the authorisation or collaboration of a doctor. But Mermet believed that the pendulum could be used to diagnose not merely what was the matter with a patient, but also what remedy would be most effective; and he described how experiments with plants had convinced him that some were more effective than conventional remedies, as doctors who had used them had found : they had obtained remarkable cures even in cancer cases. If a medically unqualified radiesthetist chose to use the pendulum in this way, obviously he would be tempted to by-pass the medical profession. Any herbalist, or homeopath, could set himself up as a curer of any and all disorders. Radiesthesia remained suspect. A few doctors practised it by themselves, or collaborated with Mermet; but in general it provoked ridicule.

THE 'BLACK BOX'

Mermet's pendulum tended to arouse amused scepticism: the reaction to Albert Abrams' version of radiesthesia was of intense and often violent hostility.

Born in America in 1863, Abrams had qualified there before going to Europe to study under Virchow, Wasserman and Helmholz; and when he returned to practise in San Francisco he already had a reputation as a neurologist, which he proceeded to enhance (he was to be described by the physician, Sir James Barr, a Vice-President of the British Medical Association, as 'by far the greatest genius the medical profession has produced for half-a-century'). His particular ability was to detect phenomena which other doctors missed; and on one occasion, while percussing a patient, he realised that the sound he heard altered according to the direction in which the patient was facing.

'Percussion' – tapping the body with a finger, or a small hammer, to aid diagnosis by enabling the doctor to pick up the vibrations, or sounds – had first been used in the 1750's by the Austrian, Leopold Auenbrugger; having employed it as a way of detecting how much wine was in his innkeeper-father's casks, Auenbrugger had realised its potential value in finding out what was happening within a patient's chest. Like many another innovator he did not live to see his idea accepted by the profession; it was taken up only in the early years of the nineteenth century. It then became, along with auscultation – listening with a stethescope's help – part of the doctor's standard diagnostic equipment. Nobody, however, had previously realised that the sound, or vibrations, might vary according to the point of the compass towards which the patient was facing.

Dangerously close though this was to occultism, it might just have proved acceptable to orthodoxy if Abrams had contented himself with demonstrating its diagnostic significance in determining what was the matter with a patient. But it led him on to experiment; and by a path curiously similar to that followed by Mermet (though Abrams was approaching the same subject from the opposite, scientific, direction) he found that it was possible to produce the same sound as he had obtained when he percussed a patient suffering from a tumour, if he percussed the body of a healthy subject who was holding, or in close contact with, a piece of diseased tissue. Further experiment convinced him that if he rigged up the equivalent of an electric circuit (though without a source of electricity), it was possible to register a 'bio-current;' and with the help of variable resistances placed within the circuit he could detect whether the diseased tissue held by the healthy individual at a point in the circuit was tuberculous, or cancerous, or whatever it might be. 'The beginning of the disease,' he explained, 'is a disturbance of electronic equilibrium within the molecule'; and with the help of another inventor he produced an instrument, the oscilloclast, which could provide a diagnosis from a piece of tissue or a drop of blood without the need for the patient to be present. It worked just as well, he claimed, if the patient were in Europe as in his California surgery.

Any chance which Abrams might have had of persuading his colleagues that his methods worked was effectively destroyed by the appearance of the oscilloclast. Although it looked as if it were designed to work on some electro-magnetic principle there was no battery, and no current; so the 'black box', as it soon came to be called, appeared to be a confidence trick. The fact that Abrams made and sold the boxes, too, was held against him (though in fact this was more to protect his discovery than to make money; he was a very wealthy man); he and his invention were savaged in the *Scientific American*. When the boxes reached Britain in the 1920's the publicity they attracted predictably annoyed the medical Establishment: but they also offered what appeared to be an ideal opportunity to demonstrate the wisdom of the decision not to give way to the clamour for formal recognition of Herbert Barker. Here, surely, was an example of precisely the kind of quackery from which the public should be protected! And in 1924 a committee of scientists was set up under Sir Thomas – later, Lord – Horder, to investigate 'the electronic reactions of Abrams'.

The report of the enquiry was communicated by Lord Horder to a meeting at the Royal Society of Medicine, and published in the *British Medical Journal* and the *Lancet* on 24th January, 1925. In sponsoring the investigation, Horder said, the Society had 'shown no little courage, since you have risked the censure of those – and they are neither few nor insubstantial – in whose nostrils the subject has an odour which is quite unsavoury'. In Horder's view this suspicion had been justified, as Abrams had made claims which were supported by the slenderest evidence, couched in jargon often associated with charlatanry; and he had gone into the business of selling his equipment. Still, the possibility could not be ignored that Abrams might have made a discovery of real scientific importance, which he had wished to exploit for gain. The committee had accordingly decided to give an exponent of Abram's technique, W. E. Boyd – a homeopathic doctor from Glasgow – a fair trial.

Boyd's instrument, which he called an 'emanometer', was not quite the same as Abrams'; but this was unimportant, as the committee's concern was clearly to show that no machine built on the same principle could work. After some preliminary experiments a test was held. Boyd and his assistants were given a succession of objects – tissues, or chemicals, 'indistinguishable by visual or other normal standards' to identify; and of twenty-five successive trials Horder had to admit, 'all were successful. The chance of this result being by accident is one in 33,554,432'.

To sceptics, so remarkable a success rate could only have been accomplished by some ingenious fraud; and this gave the committee an excuse to decide that it would be unfair to its member who had carried out the test, Whately Smith from the Air Ministry, if the report had to rest on his testimony. There must be a further test. Dr E. J. Dingwall, who then and for the next half-century was the leading expert in the detection of forms of trickery, and who was employed by the Society for Psychical Research to provide its members with advice in investigations of mediums and paranormal phenomena, was brought in as adviser. A fresh and more stringently controlled series of tests was carried out by the committee under his supervision; yet Boyd's success rate, Horder admitted, was no less impressive. The committee had consequently been left with no alternative but to accept that certain substances, when placed in the relationship Boyd indicated to his emanometer, 'produced beyond any reasonable doubt changes in the abdominal wall of "the subject" of a kind which may be detected by percussion'. Abrams' fundamental proposition, in short, had been 'established to a very high degree of probability'; and although Horder emphasised that it would be premature even to hazard a guess how it worked, and unwise to assume its reliability in the diagnosis or treatment of illness, it merited further research.

Forty years before, when the young Pierre Janet had described how it was possible to put a woman into the hypnotic state at a distance of half a mile, his Salpêtrière audience had sat in silent stupefaction. It was the same at the meeting of the Royal Society of Medicine; and when the chairman tactfully asked whether members would prefer to discuss the subject then, or on some later occasion, the audience, the *British Medical Journal's* correspondent observed, showed 'no enthusiasm' for either alternative. Many of them must have come hoping for, and expecting, a devastating exposure of chicanery. If they had been showered with cold water on entering the Society's premises they could hardly have been more taken aback.

It was not just that the investigators had found that the Abrams' electronic reaction worked, which would have been bad enough. They had also had to confess that they could find no rational explanation. And even if Boyd and his assistant had been able to get up some ingenious trick between themselves this would not explain how Horder and one of the other investigators, when themselves acting the part of the healthy catalyst, 'could definitely feel an alteration in the abdominal muscles as specimens were inserted or withdrawn through the hatch, without their knowledge'.

Years later Beverley Nichols, who happened to have read about the investigation, found himself sitting next to Horder at some function. Why, he asked, as Horder had recommended further research, had he never followed it up? A little shamefacedly, Horder admitted that it was something he ought to have done. But the reason, in retrospect, is obvious. To investigate any practice which for orthodoxy has 'an odour which is unsavoury' carries a measure of risk. If the investigator can expose it as false or fraudulent, he will win some credit. If he can show not just that it works but *how* it works, so long as it is in terms acceptable to medical science, he may win a Nobel Prize. But if he has to admit that he is unable to fathom how it works, he has given a hostage to occultism, and a boost to unqualified practitioners. One such mistake may be forgiven; but for Horder to have pursued the matter might well have blocked the way to his ultimate destination: a peerage, and a royal appointment as Physician to the King.

As a result black boxes continued to be bought and operated mainly by medically unqualified practitioners. Any doctor who used one ordinarily was careful not to let his colleagues know of his eccentricity. And ironically, Abram's theory soon had to be abandoned. The Horder committee had in one respect been justified in their initial scepticism; Boyd's manometer was, in a sense, a fetish – a ju-ju, capable of nothing unless some unexplained, perhaps psychic, current was fed into the circuit. Whatever current, vibrations, or emanations Abrams and Boyd had been picking up, they were not electro-magnetic.

Yet the fact was that the method had worked, and spectacularly well, in the Horder tests. One of Abrams' disciples in California, Ruth Drown, decided to construct a box of a different kind, in which the dials were attached to a sheet of rubber on a metal plate. Stroking the rubber with her finger, she found that at some point, when the dials were being turned, the rubber would become 'tacky' to the touch; and by experiments similar to those which Abrams had devised, she satisfied herself that by putting a spot of a patient's blood on the instrument, stroking the rubber, and manipulating the dials, the nature of the patient's illness could be diagnosed.

There was a curious similiarity, though it was not realised at the time, between the new black box and the 'rubbing-board oracle' which Edward Evans-Pritchard, later to be the Professor of Anthropology at Oxford, found in use among the Azande tribe in the course of his field work with them in Sudan in the early 1930's. It consisted of a couple of pieces of wood which the diviner would rub together, saying 'Rubbing-board, if you would speak the truth, stick'; when he asked questions the two pieces of wood answered them by continuing to slide over each other for 'no', by sliding less smoothly for 'not sure', and by sticking for 'yes'. But such was the craving for an objective diagnostic technique that some of the users of the new-style black box declined to accept that all they were doing was tapping unexplained psychic or intuitive forces. Others, however, realised that the black box must simply be a more elaborate, and potentially a more accurate, version of the radiesthetist's pendulum, and in the 1930's the two schools, Mermet's and Abrams', began to merge. Both began to describe themselves as radiesthetists, the term 'radionics' being coined initially to describe the study of the forces which made the pendulum swing, or the rubber become tacky, though it later was applied to the use of devices like the 'box'.

For Mermet, the explanation was telepathy. The spot of blood served simply as a telephone exchange, to link the two minds, radiesthetist's and patient's, much as a map could link the mind of a dowser to an underground stream. It was a matter of vibrations: the process, 'which has long been regarded as a dangerous and mysterious occult phenomenon, is nothing but a physical and natural function'. And by this time the work of J. B. Rhine and his colleagues at Duke University was providing evidence to confirm the reality of telepathy and clairvoyance. But orthodox scientists would not accept Rhine's evidence unless and until a more acceptable explanation than 'vibrations' could be found to account for the ability of two minds to communicate at a distance. As none was forthcoming, radionics and radiesthesia – and telepathy – remained outsiders.

SUGGESTION AND AUTO-SUGGESTION

So did hypnotism, as a method of treating illness. A few stage hypnotists continued to demonstrate it night after night in music halls, and in big cities a hypnotist or two were usually to be found offering their services to cure rheumatism and other disorders which the profession was by this time finding it notoriously hard to treat; but very few doctors employed it. Yet the effect of the brief period during the 1880's when it had appeared to be establishing itself as a clinical aid had not been entirely dissipated. The demonstrators of that era, in the Salpêtrière and in Nancy, had attracted onlookers who developed their own techniques out of what they had learned. And in the years between the wars hypnotism, which had had such little influence on orthodox medicine, began to seep back in ways unacceptable to the profession.

While still in his twenties, Freud had fallen under Charcot's spell in the course of a visit to Paris. Charcot, he wrote, was 'tremendously stimulating', no other human being had ever affected him in such a way, though 'whether the seed will ever bring forth fruit I do not know'. It did. Fascinated by what he had seen Freud went to Nancy, where he witnessed 'the moving spectacle of old Liébeault working among the poor women and children of the labouring classes'. He also attended Bernheim's clinics, receiving 'the profoundest impression of the possibility that there could be powerful mental processes which nevertheless remain hidden from the consciousness of man'. It was these visits, coupled with his observation of his friend Breuer's use of hypnosis in treating a hysteric patient, which were to lure Freud away from straightforward neurology, and set him on the road that was to culminate in the introduction of psycho-analysis.

Freud, though, was a doctor and a scientist; and although his emphasis on the sexual origin of hysteria and the neuroses was to lead to his being regarded as heterodox by most members of the medical profession, throughout his life he worked within its confines. His ideas, modified and expanded by disciples, eventually permeated alternative medicine; but that was to be a gradual process whose effects did not become fully apparent until after his death. Another visitor to Nancy in the 1880's was destined to make a greater, if transient, impact in the 1920's: Emile Coué, a chemist from the French town of Troyes.

As a pharmacy student Coué had come to realise that some patients felt better after taking medicines which he knew to be coloured water; and after he had the opportunity to watch Liébeault at work he began to understand why. From his experience – and in France, the local chemist was often, in effect, the local doctor – Coué came to the conclusion that the therapeutic force was exercised by the patient, not by the hypnotist, through auto-suggestion. It followed that there should be no need for the hypnotist, if people could learn to exploit their own auto-suggestive capabilities: a secular version, in other words, of Christian Science.

For this purpose, Coué found, it was no use people trying to 'will' themselves better. What they needed to do was *imagine* themselves better. As an example he pointed out how easy it is to walk along on a plank thirty centimetres wide if it is lying on the ground; but only a trained circus performer is likely to be able to walk along such a plank if it is two hundred metres *above* the ground. Willing oneself to walk along it, in such circumstances, is no help, because the imagination infects the mind with the risks of such an enterprise. But if the imagination can be persuaded that there is no risk – as in the case of sleepwalkers, who can perform terrifying balancing feats without a qualm – the plank can be walked without difficulty, whatever its height.

Coué was able to cite many such examples, some of them of more immediate application to health. Nobody, he pointed out, can will his saliva to flow; but anybody can make it flow by conjuring up a mental picture of some particularly mouth-watering dish. Logically, then, the process of digestion must depend upon the imagination to set the gastric juices, as well as the saliva, flowing. The will 'must not intervene in the practice of auto-suggestion,' he concluded. 'What we have to work for is the education of the imagination.'

To educate it, Coué went back to the ancient art of incantation. What everybody should do, he suggested, was repeat the formula 'Every day, in every way, I'm getting better and better.' Where people were suffering from some particular symptom, this could be varied, 'Every moment, the pain is passing off' – or whatever it might be. And Couéism caught on to a remarkable extent. Not just in France, but throughout the world, people tried in out in the bath or on the bus. It rivalled crosswords and Mah Jong, as one of the crazes of the bright young things (and of their parents) in the twenties. But as a craze Couéism could hardly be expected to survive (though crosswords, the opium of the commuter, have defied the passage of time). In any case most of the people who used the formula did so under the impression, never having read Coué's instructions, that it was a way of willing themselves better. So far as most doctors were concerned it was no more than a rather silly game; and during the great depression of the early 1930's it quietly faded out.

CAYCE

Along with Freud and Coué there was one other individual with a remarkable reputation in the years between the wars who owed it initially to the surge of interest there had been in hypnotism in the 1880's. Edgar Cayce, born in 1877 in Christian County, Kentucky, was from earliest childhood psychic: a freak, as he often thought of himself. Before he could read he could describe historical events as if he had witnessed them. At school, though in some respects a hopeless dunce, he could occasionally reel off the answers to questions from books he had never read. Voices in his inner ear periodically guided him; sometimes he enjoyed second sight; and he would give a diagnosis, when he was ill, of what was the matter with him by talking in his sleep.

As a young man, Cayce mysteriously lost his voice, so that he could not speak above a whisper; and treatment by a hypnotist, though while he was in the trance he could speak as well as before, did not restore his voice when he came out of the trance. But he had a neighbour, Al Layne, who had become an osteopath by the dubious route of a mail order course, and who had then studied hypnosis by the same method. It occurred to Layne that what Cayce needed was not straightforward suggestion under hypnosis. Instead it should be suggested to him under hypnosis that he should take over, and prescribe whatever was right for himself. The method worked; Cayce's voice was restored.

Not merely did it work for Cayce himself; Layne found that Cayce in his trances could also diagnose and prescribe for the illnesses of others. Layne would hypnotise him; Cayce would then explain what was the matter with people who came to him – though he neither saw them, nor knew who they were, as Layne would hypnotise him before they came into his room. And soon Cayce's reputation was made when he diagnosed that a child who was choking to death had a button in her windpipe, something that the X-rays had missed, because it was made of celluloid.

For the rest of his life Cayce was to give these 'readings'. At first he took no fees, so that he could not be accused of practising medicine; and he did not court publicity. But his record was striking; hundreds of case histories remain, many of them well-documented and attested, of readings he gave which later were found to be correct. Sceptics sometimes tried to expose him – among them Muensterburg, Professor of Psychology at Harvard, who characteristically declined to publish his findings when he was unable to detect any deception. Unable to proceed against him for practising medicine, because he did not accept payment, the New York authorities arrested him and his household on a charge of fortune-telling; but the judge ruled that whatever Cayce might be doing it was not that. Although eventually he was persuaded to charge for readings the amount remained modest – as, by all accounts, he himself did. But neither before nor since has there been such a wealth of recorded evidence about the ability of a healer – or, as Cayce preferred to call himself, a 'psychic diagnostician'.

ORTHODOXY

There were many other healers, though, in this period, as indeed there have been in every period. How then did the medical profession manage to avoid being brought into discredit by its manifest incompetence? Considering the great advances there had been in medical knowledge, orthodox medical *treatment* in the 1920's in some respects reached its nadir.

As soon as the First World War ended, and there was no further need for diagnoses like 'shell-shock', orthodox medicine reverted to its old division of diseases into organic and functional. There was, however, a further modification. Having come into use as a handy way to explain those symptoms for which no physical cause could be found, 'functional' now became even more suspect. There must be *some* physical cause, purists felt; so medical students were taught that functional really meant 'NYD' – Not Yet Diagnosed.

To replace it increasing use was made of the suffix '-itis'. It meant no more than 'inflamed'; but a patient who was told he had gastritis felt relieved, under the impression that his stomach trouble had been diagnosed – and the doctor felt relieved of the need to find out why it had begun in the first place. In particular 'colitis' – inflammation of the colon – enjoyed a vogue as a diagnosis. Toxic substances in the intestines, doctors explained, were responsible for a great variety of symptoms, from gout to nettlerash; and soon it displaced 'functional' as the conventional explanation for any disorder which could not be accounted for. It was all the more financially valuable to the profession because tracts of intestines could be removed by surgery without doing patients much harm; and countless patients underwent the operations as a consequence.

By an extraordinary example of nature imitating art, during the 1920's a medical fashion arose which might have been borrowed straight out of *The Doctor's Dilemma*. Shaw's 'machine-made and beeswaxed' London surgeon, Cutler Walpole, had decided that the reason for illness was blood-poisoning ('ninety-five percent of the human race suffer from it'); and that the cause of blood-poisoning was the 'nuciform sac' ('your nuciform sac is full of decaying matter – undigested food and waste products – rank ptomaines.'). All that was needed to restore health, therefore, was a simple piece of surgery, to take the sac out. The 1920's version took only a slightly different form: 'focal infection'. The focus of infection might be in the gut, which could be cut out, or in the teeth, which could be extracted, or in any part of the body which could be removed without excessive risk; and hundreds of thousands, perhaps millions, of people were operated upon so that the focus could be found (often – again to echo Cutler Walpole – none could be traced) and excised, for as many guineas as the surgeon felt the patient could afford.

It did not take long for 'focal sepsis' to fall into disrepute among those members of the profession who were not committed to it. But 'There is a fashion in operations as there is in sleeves and skirts,' Shaw had observed in his preface; the triumph of a surgeon who makes a previously dangerous operation reasonably safe 'is usually followed by a rage for that operation, not only among the doctors but actually among the patients'. So it turned out to be with operations for focal sepsis. The psychiatrist William Sargant has recently recalled that when he went as a medical student to St Mary's in the late 1920's, hundreds of teeth were still being needlessly extracted by Sir William Wilcox on the grounds that they harboured focal sepsis; and one of the students' jobs as assistants at the operations was to try to explain to patients 'why their good teeth had to come out when Sir William's filthy teeth stayed in'. Then, and for many years to come, the operation 'made large fortunes for several members of the staff; staff members were even elected bcause of their work in it, and stayed on working at it for years after it was discredited'.

'All professions are conspiracies against the laity,' Shaw's Sir Patrick Cullen had remarked; and here was a prime example, as few voices were publicly raised against the procedure. Only a few doctors, too, stood out against the exclusively physiological interpretation of disease; notably the German physician Georg Groddeck, with his insistence that the unconscious mind not merely can be the cause of symptoms, but can also dictate the form they take, so that a sore throat may represent an inability to 'swallow' some situation like an impending visit from mother-in-law, and backache an intimation that something is going on which the patient 'cannot stand'. Freud was attracted to Groddeck's interpretation but this did Groddeck's thesis little service, so long as Freud's theories were anathema.

In England, F. G. Crookshank sarcastically observed that the way things were going made him wonder why 'some hard-boiled and orthodox clinician does not describe emotional weeping as a new disease, calling it paroxysmal lachrymation, and suggesting treatment by belladonna, astringent local application, avoidance of sexual excess, tea, tobacco and alcohol, and a salt-free diet with restriction of fluid intake; proceeding in the event of failure to early removal of the tear glands'. But Crookshank was a maverick: he even preached the heresy that microbes did not cause disease (to blame them, he argued, was like blaming bullets for causing wars; what needed to be discovered was why wars broke out); and his works reached only a tiny audience.

Most doctors felt in loyalty bound not to foul the nest, even with the aim of preventing their colleagues from fouling it. Some doctors, too, ran their own rackets, of the kind A. J. Cronin was to describe in *The Citadel*, and which he owned up to in his autobiographical *Adventures in Two Worlds*. As a young doctor, Cronin confessed, he had made his reputation and the beginnings of his fortune by the treatment he gave for 'asthenia' (the prefix 'neur' had been quietly dropped, as nervous disorders were dangerously close to the psychiatric, rather than the physiological, camp). Whenever patients complaining of a feeling of weakness, lassitude or malaise came to Cronin, instead of giving them one of the standard tonics (which he knew to be useless) by the bottle he gave the same tonic by hypodermic syringe. His injections for asthenia, he recalled, became 'as much the mode, and as eagerly sought after, as Manuel's new spring gowns. Again and again, my sharp and shining needle sank into fashionable buttocks, bared upon the finest linen sheets.' And this 'hocus-pocus' – for he was under no illusions that the tonic itself would be any more effective by this route than when swallowed – often had the desired result because, he decided, it gave his patients, and particularly the 'bored and languid women', a renewed interest in life. So did the cost: 'My treatment would never have been deemed worthwhile had I not charged for it an appropriately exorbitant fee.'

One reason Cronin and his colleagues were able to get away with it was to be discovered as the result of an experiment undertaken at a London hospital and reported in the *Quarterly Journal of Medicine* in 1933. Two cardiologists, William Evans and C. Hoyle, had found that the effect of pain-relieving drugs such as morphine appeared to show considerable variation in the treatment of cases of angina; and not all patients tolerated them well, apart from the risk of addiction. There must be some subjective element, they decided, influencing patients' reactions; and they decided to try an experiment of the kind which has since come to be known as 'controlled'. Instead of simply testing the new treatment on a group of patients, they divided the patients up into two groups, giving the routine pain-killer to one group and the new drug to the other, to compare the effects.

The new drug was not, in fact, new; it was bicarbonate of soda. The results were striking: thirty-eight per cent of the patients who took the bicarbonate of soda, believing it to be a pain-killer, were satisfactorily relieved of their pain. That this was no fluke was to be demonstrated the same year in another experiment in which the symptoms of one-third of a group of patients with common colds cleared up when they were given lactose – milk-sugar. As both bicarbonate of soda and lactose could be considered 'pharmacologically inert' for the purposes of the experiments, the obvious explanation, soon to be confirmed by further trials, was that where the treatment was successful it must be because the patient's expectation had in some way influenced the outcome: in other words, through auto-suggestion.

After years of deriding Couéism and dismissing hypnotism, the medical profession could not be expected to accept this as exciting evidence of the mind's power over the body; unless, again, some plausible neurological explanation had been presented, perhaps of the kind that had been offered by Braid and Carpenter. 'Heightened sensitivity,' however, hardly fitted the fresh evidence. So the symptom-removing properties of bicarbonate of soda and lactose were attributed to 'placebo effect'. The term placebo, the Latin for 'I will please' had been in use for centuries to describe any medicine which had no medicinal ingredients; coloured water, say, of the kind sold as hair restorer by peddlers at country fairs. Placebos had been known to cure but the orthodox assumption had been that the people they cured had not really been ill: they had only imagined they were ill. That angina patients only imagined that they were in pain, or that people with the usual symptoms of heavy colds had somehow managed to mimic them, was hardly conceivable. Still, as some explanation had to be found which would save the medical profession from the embarrassing need to re-admit the mind as one of the chief influences in promoting recovery, placebo-effect was hurriedly pressed into service. Patients who recovered after placebo treatment, the implication was, could not have been really ill, even if their symptoms had been real.

Doctors did not know it, or if they did they would certainly not have admitted it, but the success of most of their treatments in this period could be attributed almost entirely to auto-suggestion. With a handful of exceptions the medicines in common use still had little, if any, intrinsic value. Few advances in treatment were made in the 1920's other than the introduction of insulin for diabetics and liver extract for anaemia – palliatives rather than cures. The chief advantage, in fact, so far as patients were concerned was the decline of doctors' confidence in purgings and bleedings. But the public did not realise this, any more than they realised that the incidence of mortality from infectious diseases, which continued to fall, was the result less of improved immunisation procedures or drugs than of improved sanitation, hygiene, and nourishment. So the medical profession managed to survive with its image reasonably unscarred.

It had no serious rivals in this period. Homeopathy no longer gave cause for concern, in spite of the fact that it had risen in the social world. Queen Mary had been brought up in a family treated by a homeopath: her second son, the Duke of York, became a believer in homeopathy; and in the 1920's John Weir, Professor of Materia Medica at the London School of Homeopathy, was appointed physician to the Royal

Family. The appointment caused wry amusement, rather than wrath, in the medical profession; and Weir was soon enveloped in respectability, with a knighthood in 1932 and, in the same year, offers to lecture on homeopathy at the Royal Society of Medicine and at the British Medical Association's centenary gathering. His rise reflected homeopathy's decline. It was respectable to go to a homeopath; but it was no longer adventurous.

Orthodoxy lost ground only to the manipulators. In the United States osteopathy continued to expand, and to win formal recognition. In the process, though, osteopaths began to rely on more conventional methods of treatment, even on drugs; and to regard themselves as more akin to the medical profession than to the chiropractors (one of them described chiropractic in 1925 as 'a malignant tumor on the body of osteopathy'). A few chiropractors were tempted to move in the same direction, in the hope of securing official recognition; but the most influential of them, B. J. Palmer – son of the founder – held to his father's creed. He believed in the existence of what he described as 'innate intelligence', centred in the brain, and influenced by 'universal intelligence'; these being the decisive forces in health and disease. This in no way diminished the importance of manipulation; it merely shifted the manipulator's focus of attention from the lower back to the neck. To B. J. Palmer the first and second cervical vertebrae, as 'the vital intermediate space between brain and body', were where obstruction was most likely to occur, producing 'starvation of forces or energies made for the body, but not reaching the body'. Couched though it was in mechanist terms, this was clearly a vitalist belief; and in the years between the wars many chiropractors suffered for Palmer's vigorously proclaimed heresies, prosecutions for the illicit practice of medicine often subjecting them to fines and jail sentences.

There were too few chiropractors in Britain to alarm the medical Establishment; but it was roused to action in the early 1930's by an attempt to secure legislative recognition for osteopathy. When a parliamentary committee of enquiry was set up to look into the proposal, the Royal Colleges and the British Medical Association joined forces against it; and they successfully exposed the deficiencies of the British School of Osteopathy – deficiencies chiefly the result of the refusal of the General Medical Council to allow any co-operation with osteopaths. The committee's verdict was that the osteopaths would have to put their school in better order, before they could hope to achieve the status they were seeking. Its report, though, was critical of the training of osteopaths, rather than of manipulation as such; and in 1936 there was what looked as if it might be a decisive breakthrough, when Herbert Barker was called out of retirement to give a demonstration of his technique at St Thomas's Hospital.

Although Barker had never claimed to be anything but a bonesetter, his technique when dealing with the spine resembled that of the osteopaths; they could feel manipulation was also on trial. He treated eighteen patients who had not responded to orthodox methods; and after sufficient time had elapsed to assess whether the effects were lasting, ten were pronounced cured and five improved. In a leading article the *Times* urged the need for further demonstrations; if they confirmed the value of manipulation 'steps ought to be taken at once to make such teaching as widely available as possible not only to British surgeons, but to surgeons in all parts of the world'. Facilities were later made available for Barker to be filmed while demonstrating his technique; and this, too, the *Times* welcomed. 'Thanks to these films all future generations will be able to avail themselves of a body of knowledge and experience of which so many in this present generation are the beneficiaries' – among them, the writer noted, being the Duke of Kent, Earl Beatty, John Galsworthy, Lord Hawke and Georges Carpentier. 'The battle for manipulative surgery is won,' Barker delightedly claimed. But a few weeks later Hitler's forces moved into Poland; and by the time the war ended Barker and his techniques were only a hazy memory.

Chapter Five

THE PHARMACOLOGICAL REVOLUTION

The Second World War witnessed a transformation in medical treatment of a kind unparalleled in history, and unlikely to be repeated. For twenty years after Ehrlich's 'magic bullet', Salvarsan, had been introduced no successor could be found; and in *Man and Medicine*, published in 1931, Henry Sigerist felt compelled to admit that although there had been massive advances in medical knowledge, they had done little to improve medical treatment. A few months later, however, the chemist, Gerhard Domagk, working for I. G. Farben discovered that streptoccocal infections in laboratory animals could be controlled by a dyestuff, 'prontosil red'; and shortly before the war the first of the 'sulpha drugs', 'M and B', came on the market. For the first time doctors could actually treat and cure meningitis, pneumonia and other disorders, as distinct from helplessly observing their progress from the bedside. Penicillin, brought into production during the war, proved even more effective and safer than the sulpha drugs; streptomycin followed, speeding up the fall in the mortality rate from TB; and in the late 1940's the arrival of the 'broad spectrum' antibiotics – chloramphenicol, aureomycin and terramycin – meant that Erhlich's concept became obsolescent. They were not so much bullets as grape-shot, lethal to a wide range of pathogenic bacteria.

Unorthodox forms of medical treatment consequently began to seem irrelevant, particularly in Britain, after the National Health Service had been set up in 1948. Shaw had not been alone in his belief that it was crazy for doctors to be paid by people who were ill instead of being paid to keep people well; Socialists had long argued that medical treatment should be free – paid for, that is, out of taxation, or from some all-embracing national insurance scheme. It would take time, the Labour Government explained, for the backlog of ill-health to be cleared. Children who had grown up in slums might be suffering from calcium deficiency, say, or decayed teeth; for a while the profession would have to concentrate on the eradication of sickness. But in due course the NHS would become, as its name indicated, a national *health* service, with prevention of disease as its primary function.

THE NATIONAL HEALTH SERVICE

At last the dream of the French revolutionaries appeared to be on the verge of fulfilment. Disease, they had believed, was largely the reflection of a sick society. 'Living in the midst of ease, surrounded by the pleasures of life,' the Girondin Lanthénas had written of the aristos in 1792, 'their irascible pride, their bitter spleen, their abuses and the excess to which their contempt of all principles leads them, make them a prey to infirmities of every kind'; whereas the virtuous poor only needed to be better nourished, better housed, and provided with better facilities for enjoying fresh air and exercise, to enjoy good health. The proposition had become integral to left-wing thought. Nor could it readily be dismissed as a Socialist pipe dream: common sense suggested that as living standards rose the incidence of diseases associated with poverty, over-crowding and under-nourishment must decline, leaving the medical profession more time to concentrate on finding ways to prevent the disorders of affluence. In his own self-interest, surely, every doctor would want to show patients on his list how to keep well. The healthier they became the less work he would be called upon to do.

Although the medical profession regarded the proposed Health Service as a threat, and fiercely resisted it, their fears centred around the possibility that the State would convert doctors into civil servants, and exercise more control over them by restricting their right to prescribe the drugs they believed most suitable, regardless of cost. The then Minister for Health, Aneurin Bevan, went out of his way to remove their apprehensions. But in doing so, the herbalists realised when the Bill was going through Parliament, he would reinforce the profession's monopoly.

Herbalists had been hard hit during the nineteenth century by the discovery of ways in which to extract alkaloids from plants – quinine from cinchona, cocaine from the coca shrub, and several others – providing drugs which were much more effective, even if more dangerous, than herbal remedies. In the 1860's some British practitioners had made an effort to put their craft on a more specific basis by setting up the National Institute of Medical Herbalists, aiming to end the practice by which they could sell the doses they themselves prescribed, and introducing examinations. But this had caused a split, many herbalists refusing to accept the need for so drastic a change; and although the movement survived, it was on a greatly reduced scale. By the late 1940's, about the only advantage the remaining herbalists still enjoyed was that their remedies cost less than the medicines bought over the chemists' counters, and often very much less than those obtained on a doctor's prescription.

Under the NHS, medicines prescribed by a doctor would cost the patient nothing; and the herbalists, alarmed, asked a member of parliament to put their case for inclusion before the Minister. Bevan's reply was that they must set their house in order before their case could even be considered. This did not merely mean that they would have to settle their differences, and set up a single organisation with a training scheme and qualifications of a kind which would meet with the Ministry's approval. It carried the further implication that if their reorganisation was deemed satisfactory, they might be admitted to the NHS, but only on the same basis as other medical auxiliaries. They would then, like physiotherapists, come largely under the direction of the medical profession, accepting only such patients as doctors chose to send them.

Naturally this was not what the herbalists wanted. Their remedies were not designed to complement the drugs which the pharmaceutical industry was now pouring out, but to render them unnecessary. Few doctors would accept this; very few would even consider prescribing herbs. So the herbalists elected not to try to enter the NHS; and a hard time they were to have of it for the next few years. Yet they won little public sympathy, as the general impression was that they were expendable. Doubtless there would continue to be a small market for some of their wares – old-fashioned ladies wanting old-fashioned remedies, and gullible folk looking for an elixir (and for some quack to provide it). But surely such superstitions would gradually die out?

Nature cure practitioners – naturopaths, as they now styled themselves – were in a slightly less vulnerable position, as it was their services rather than their remedies that they had to sell; and this also applied to healers, radiesthetists and hypnotists. But these groups had no prospect of qualifying for admission to the NHS. The only other medically-unqualified practitioners who had to make up their minds whether to apply to join the health service, or risk deprivation outside it, were the osteopaths and chiropractors.

In the United States they had less to worry about. In most States of the Union osteopaths had become to all intents doctors, with the same rights and privileges as members of the medical profession, and trained in many orthodox techniques. (When, in 1959, a committee investigated osteopathy on behalf of the American Medical Association, it reported that the standards of entry into, and qualification from, osteopathic training schools was as high as in medical schools, and higher than some). Chiropractic, too, though still unrecognised in a few States, was beginning to catch up. And as in many parts of the country chiropractors still provided the only medical services in the districts where they practised, when they were proceeded against for practising medicine without the requisite qualifications or for illegally dispensing drugs, sympathetic juries often refused to convict.

In Britain, osteopaths (there were still very few chiropractors) were more vulnerable. Unlike the United States, the great majority of their patients came to them to be treated for backache and associated symptoms like sciatica and rheumatism. During the war the belief had grown that the majority of cases of backache were caused by a 'slipped disc' – by one of the shock absorbers between the vertebrae protruding and impinging upon a nerve; and this had meant that osteopaths had lost many potential patients to surgeons. And 1949 saw the introduction of cortisone, which for a time looked as though it might be the answer to orthodoxy's prayers. Not merely did cortisone enable patients who had long been crippled by spinal trouble to leave their beds, walk and even run: it broke fresh ground by being the first of the new drugs to be effective against a degenerative disease, as distinct from an infection.

Might it not be the precursor of many others, as 'M & B' had been of the antibiotics? If so medicine would be even more strikingly transformed, as the incidence of most of the infectious diseases had already been greatly reduced even before the wonder drugs appeared, whereas rhumatism, cancer, heart attacks and other disorders arising out of premature ageing or faulty metabolism were, if anything, on the increase.

PSYCHOSOMATIC MEDICINE

There was, however, a vitalist spectre at the feast. Medical scientists had continued to assert that organic disease could only arise from some physical or chemical cause: germ, virus or toxin. They had paid no attention to Groddeck, or his disciples. In 1937 a Scots doctor, J. L. Halliday, achieved the unusual feat of persuading the editor of the *British Medical Journal* to accept an article on 'psychological factors in rheumatism', in which he argued that as there was ample evidence to show that they could bring about alterations 'in chemistry, rhythm, secretion and even structure', doctors ought not to content themselves with diagnosing what was physically the matter with the patient: they ought also to look for underlying or precipitating psychological causes, asking themselves what kind of a person he was, why he fell ill at that particular time and if he had any reason for falling ill, because the answer might provide useful diagnostic clues. Such theorising, though, had been dismissed as speculative. It was more difficult for the profession to ignore the implications of an ingenious piece of research by two New York doctors, Stewart Wolf and Harold G. Wolff.

In their *Human Gastric Function*, published in 1943, Wolf and Wolff described how they had decided to take advantage of an unusual opportunity which had presented itself to observe the digestive process in action. 'Tom', a janitor at their hospital, had obstructed his gullet as a child and for the remainder of his life had to be fed through a tube inserted into his digestive tract. This, they realised, gave them the same opportunity which had been exploited over a century before by a Canadian, William Beaumont, who in the course of treating a trapper for a bullet wound in his stomach had watched the progress of different kinds of food and drink as they passed the site of the wound. On one occasion, when the trapper was angry, the food on its way through his stomach was tinged with yellow bile; the explanation, Beaumont surmised, must be that the arousal of the emotion had influenced the action of his gastric juices. Wolf and Wolff decided to see what effect an emotional upset would have on 'Tom'. While they were observing what was happening in his digestive system, they casually commiserated with him on losing his job. His stomach lining paled from red to near white, much as people's faces do when in a state of shock; and his mucous membrane became fragile. so that the slightest friction caused it to bleed. When he was reassured, the membrane soon recovered its former condition.

There could hardly have been a clearer demonstration of the reality of what the profession had dismissed as popular myth, or folk-lore: the notion that people in stressful situations became more prone to indigestion and to stomach ulcers. And in 1947 the publication of Flanders Dunbar's *Mind and Body*, describing the research which had been carried out in this field, launched 'psychosomatic medicine', a relatively new term for doctors, as she explained, and 'a very new one to most laymen'. A New York psychiatrist, Dunbar was more influenced by Freud than by Groddeck; and her efforts to relate specific symptoms to specific personality types, and to trace back the personality types to traumas suffered in infancy, were calculated to provoke resistance within the profession. Still, her book was sufficiently well documented to impress even the reviewer on the *Journal of the American Medical*

Association; and sufficiently readable to secure healthy sales among the general public.

By the 1950's 'psychosomatic medicine' was shedding the inverted commas with which editors of medical journals had fastidiously (and sometimes satirically) enclosed it; the resistance to it within the profession proved too strong to overcome, partly because the great majority of doctors had been indoctrinated with mechanistic assumptions, partly because of the rapid development of specialist disciplines. Consultant dermatologists, say, or rheumatologists, did not as a rule relish psychological, let alone psychoanalytical, speculation about the causes of acne or arthritis. When they wrote textbooks they often warned students against diagnosing symptoms as psychosomatic unless and until every other possible physical or chemical cause had been eliminated. A few eminent members of the profession actually dismissed psychosomatic medicine as a passing fad. It was unworthy, Sir George Pickering asserted in 1950, even of consideration by medical science.

How mistaken this view had been was soon to be demonstrated by a report in the *British Medical Journal* of an experiment carried out in a London hospital. A boy had been admitted suffering from ichthyosis, most of his body being covered with a malodorous horny layer, as if it were a cluster of warts. None of the treatments tried was any use; skin grafts taken from parts of his body which were unaffected were soon as bad as the skin they had replaced. One possibility remained untried: hypnotism. An experiment carried out not long before had demonstrated the effectiveness of auto-suggestion even without hypnotism, in getting rid of warts; children suffering from them had been divided into two groups, one group receiving the then standard treatment, and the other participating in 'magic' – using pictures of the warts, drawing circles round them, and daily reducing the warts' size on paper; and the magic had worked better than the standard medical treatment. It was decided that suggestion reinforced by hypnosis should be tried on the 'rhino boy'' as by this time he was being described. Out of caution – and also to ensure that if the scales fell from his body, it really was the suggestion which was responsible – the treatment was carried out in stages. He was hypnotised, and told that a certain area of his skin would clear up; and when it did, leaving skin that was almost normal in texture, the process was repeated until recovery was complete.

As very few doctors had any experience of hypnotising patients, the way should have been open for hypnotists to take advantage of the publicity. But hypnotism had never succeeded in divesting itself of the Svengali image. Although there were probably at least as many hypnotherapists, as they called themselves, as there were herbalists, they had no effective organisation. The group which came forward to take advantage of the evidence which psychosomatic researchers were providing was, unexpectedly, the Churches Council of Healing, a body backed by all denominations in Britain except the Catholics, who in those pre-ecumenical times would not formally collaborate in such ventures.

The Council's genesis could be traced back to the end of the nineteenth century, when members of the Protestant Churches who had retained a belief in the Church's healing mission became alarmed not so much by the growing materialism of the medical profession as by the way in which Christian Science was attracting recruits: recruits, too, from the well-to-do middle classes on whose allegiance the Episcopalian Church could normally have counted. The Emmanuel Movement, founded in the early 1900s in Boston, and the Guild of Health, its London counterpart, were designed to revive the mission.

They accordingly sought the profession's co-operation. The British Medical Association politely set up a committee; but its report, though making soothing references to the valuable role of the clergy in maintaining patients' morale, insisted that all forms of healing which were designated as spiritual or psychic were attributable to suggestion, and that suggestion was effective 'only in cases of what are generally termed "functional" disorders'. It was a clear intimation that the profession did not intend to relax its rule that doctors must not allow any unqualified practitioner to *treat* patients, even if he were in holy orders; and the Guild of Health did not choose to pursue the issue further.

There were always a few churchmen who believed that the

mission should be revived, among them William Temple, who became Archbishop of Canterbury during the Second World War. Although he did not live to see it, a new organisation, the Churches' Council of Healing, was set up after the war along the lines he had planned; and in the early 1950s his successor and the Archbishop of York together named the members of a commission to investigate the subject, the aim being to assist the clergy in the exercise of healing, 'and to encourage increasing understanding and co-operation between them and the medical profession'.

It was not the Archbishops' intention, clearly, to provoke any confrontation with the profession; and one of the commission's first acts was to ask the British Medical Association to co-operate. The BMA's response was again to set up its own investigating committee; and its report, published in 1955, differed only in emphasis from the one published before the First World War. It warily admitted the possibility that spiritual ministrations might help in treating patients 'suffering from psychogenic disorders, including psychosomatic states, in which physical symptoms result from emotional disturbances,' and it conceded that 'various forms of neurosis, alcoholism and other functional disorders' ('functional' by this time being by implication a psychiatric condition) could actually be cured by religious conversion. But like its predecessor, the committee rejected claims of cures of organic disorders -- 'We have seen no evidence that there is any special type of illness cured solely by spiritual healing which cannot be cured by medical methods which do not involve such claims'; and it patronisingly suggested that the clergy or their lay helpers should confine their efforts to providing patients with 'reassurance' and 'peace of mind'.

As nearly half the members of the Archbishops' Commission were also members either of the medical profession or of its affiliates, its report – published in 1958 – could hardly be expected to reject the BMA Committee's findings. It contented itself with a mild protest that the Church's healing ministry 'cannot be completely described in terms of psychological medicine, nor can its ministry be regarded merely as an important environmental factor'; and it insisted that there was much more to healing than the BMA Committee had allowed. But it was not prepared to defy orthodoxy by reaffirming positively that organic illness *could* be cured by 'supernormal' means.

As it happened, one such cure was reported soon after the report appeared. In *The Lonely Sea and the Sky* Francis Chichester described how, suffering from lung trouble, he had been to see one of the leading surgeons in Britain, who callously exhibited him to a group of medical students, telling them in his presence that his was 'a typical case of an advanced carcinoma'. A biopsy confirmed that Chichester had cancer of the lung; and he would have submitted to be operated upon had his wife Sheila not persuaded him to refuse, taken him out of the hospital and brought him home, where he recovered.

Chichester was to attribute his recovery to his wife's 'strange and amazing flair for health and healing'. Believing as she did in the power of prayer, she had asked many people of all denominations to pray for him; and although this had caused him some embarrassment he had come to accept that the power was miraculous. In the colloquial sense, at least, it surely was; a few months later Chichester became the first yachtsman ever to make the solo crossing of the Atlantic from Plymouth to New York.

Not that Chichester's recovery would have been likely to influence the decisions of the Archbishops' Commissioners, had they still been conferring. Their medical experts would certainly have assured them that such cases, not rare, could be attributed to 'spontaneous remission'.

One important point, however, that the Commission's report did make was in connection with scientific experiments. Some witnesses had suggested that they were the only way to settle the issue whether or not healing worked; but the Commission excused itself from the responsibility on the ground that it had neither the resources nor the qualifications. 'In any case, the Commission does not think research of this kind germane to its purpose, since it could only solve the scientific problem of the connection between healing and a particular kind of intervention regarded simply as a spatio-temporal event; it could not show whether the healing was supernatural.' The reason for this caution was obvious. Irritated though many of the clerical members of the Commission must have been by the BMA's polite scepticism they were more worried by a new development on the other flank; the emergence of spirit, or spiritual, healing, as an alternative to what the clergy had usually described as faith healing.

The Churches had tended to think of faith as the essential ingredient, in the sense that it opened up the recipient to the divine grace which was bestowed upon him. Spiritualists believed in the divine grace, but they did not feel it was necessary for the recipient to have faith in it. They had begun to set up churches in the later years of the nineteenth century, but until after the Second World War the main emphasis had been on communicating with the spirits. A few individuals, though, had become healers; and among those who had given evidence to the Archbishops' Commission, supported by an impressive array of testimonials, was Harry Edwards, by that time the best-known healer in Britain, who claimed that his powers were mediated by spirit guides.

In the 1930's Edwards had been a rationalist, contemplating a career in politics; but he had been invited to go to a spiritualist séance, and heard from the mediums there that he had healing gifts. Experimenting, he found that he could indeed cure people of disorders for whom orthodox treatment had been ineffective; and healing became his full-time occupation. So far from being hostile to orthodoxy Edwards had spirit 'guides' who were orthodoxy's heroes, Pasteur and Lister; and he studied anatomy and physiology, so that he could not be accused of putting patients at risk while showing them that joints which had long been locked by rheumatoid arthritis could become flexible once more. He also introduced a course for members and prospective members of the National Federation of Spiritual Healers, designed to make them better acquainted with the history, theories and practices involved. But the course events had taken made it obvious that he, and the Federation could expect no recognition from the medical profession, and little sympathy from the hierarchy of the Established Church.

105

Spiritualism, though, could be presented as a religion (which for some spiritual healers it was); and this gave a chance for members of the Federation to carry on their work even in hospitals, however hostile the doctors might be. With management committees' consent, they could visit any patient who called for their services. As this privilege could easily have been withdrawn if the healers made it too obvious they were treating patients, as distinct from ministering to their spiritual requirements, Edwards warned them against making exhibitions of themselves in any way – for example, by going into trances. The *British Medical Journal* was not appeased. Spiritual healers, an editorial complained in 1960, had 'slipped through the guard of two hundred and thirty-five hospital management committees' by this deception, in defiance of the General Medical Council's directive that any medical practitioner who 'by his presence, advice and co-operation' knowingly assisted anybody not registered as a medical practitioner to practise medicine, was liable to erasure. Ridiculing Edwards' claims for the validity of his cures, the editorial concluded with a call to MPs to ask the Minister of Health whether it was his policy 'to admit to Britain's State hospitals healers who claim to cure disease by supernormal means': a view supported by a number of correspondents, one of whom protested that hospital committees showed 'so little confidence in their medical and surgical staffs that they have seen fit to return to the cave, by encouraging the belief in the control of man's environment by magical means', and another who claimed that all that medical science had achieved 'in the face of desperate odds' by insisting on 'the scientific method of observation and mensuration' was now in jeopardy. 'Should we allow ourselves to slip back to the hocus-pocus of medieval concepts?'

In its editorial, the *BMJ* argued that though healing might appear to be successful, the 'cures' could be accounted for by mistakes in diagnosis, spontaneous coincidental remissions, and the effects of suggestion: 'hence modern statistical devices to eliminate bias in clinical trials'. All right, then, Edwards replied: let there be trials of healing with such devices. But this, too, was unacceptable. Even when the healers offered to allow themselves to be tested without entering the hospital, by using 'absent healing' – comparable to, and often including, prayer – the project was turned down. The Cambridge psychologist R. H. Thouless, who had been a member of the Archbishops' Commission, tried to set up an experiment in which hospital patients would be divided into two matched groups, in pairs: absent healing being given to one of each pair and not the other, with neither patients nor hospital staff to know which was which until the conclusion of the experiment. But although the formal attitude of the profession was that healing did not work except by suggestion, and that consequently absent healing could not work at all, the GMC's rule against co-operation with unqualified practitioners was invoked, and the experiment blocked.

An alternative was to follow up cases where Edwards had claimed success, to find whether any of his cures were inexplicable in orthodox terms; and an attempt at this was made by a London doctor, Louis Rose, who came to the conclusion that in the cases of cancer which had been claimed as cures, none could positively be attributed to Edwards' healing. But to reach this verdict, Rose had to accept some ludicrous propositions: for example, that in a case where cancerous tissue had been found at a biopsy, and the man had subsequently been pronounced free from cancer, the cure might have been the result of the fortunate chance that all the cancerous tissue had been removed for the biopsy. In other cases, too, where there was no dispute about the cure, it could be attributed to the delayed results of earlier orthodox treatment. The only cures which the profession were prepared to accept, Edwards complained, were of patients who had never been treated by a doctor, but in such cases, as there would have been no medical history, 'you would dispute the healing because there could not have been a proper diagnosis. It's a case of heads I win, tails you lose.'

Edwards was, in fact, wasting his time trying to convince medical scientists of his ability to heal by supernatural means. Even the possibility of paranormal healing (the implied distinction being that in Edwards' case, the force was divine and consequently not, or not necessarily, material; whereas 'paranormal' left the door open for the eventual discovery of some force analogous to radiations, or magnetism) was rejected; usually without serious consideration, and sometimes with even greater violence than spiritual healing of the traditional kind, as if there were a deep fear that to contemplate a paranormal explanation would be to cast doubt on the mechanist principles of medicine – as indeed it would have been. And some of those who tried to show that there were such forces, as yet unexplained, became martyrs to their faith.

ORGONE

One of them was Wilhelm Reich. Born in Austria just before the turn of the century, Reich had become a psycho-analyst in Vienna; but he had soon broken away from Freud. Like Groddeck he felt that bodily posture often reflected emotional disturbance – 'psychological armouring'; and he came to believe that what was required was a combination of analysis and physical manipulation, to release tensions of mind and muscle. He found, though, that patients could release their own tensions, if they could enjoy orgasm; and out of this discovery he developed a theory that there was a form of bioenergy, 'orgone' – similar to Mesmer's animal magnetism, as orgone existed in the atmosphere, but could be accumulated and stored and then utilised for various purposes, including healing. According to the nature of their disorders patients could be treated by a tube coming from an orgone box and aimed at whatever organ was giving them trouble; or they could sit for a while in an orgone box and absorb the energy.

In 1950 Reich, by this time working in laboratories at Oranur in the United States, decided to see whether orgone could be used to counteract the effects of radiation; and he began experiments with small amounts of radium. The results were startling: it was as if the radium and the orgone fed on each other, producing a violent reaction, the fall-out producing 'the Oranur sickness', killing off the laboratory mice and causing leukemia-like symptoms in some of the laboratory workers. In the end, however, the orgone level appeared to return to normal, as if satisfied with what it had accomplished.

'It runs mad, runs berserk,' Reich concluded, but if given the opportunity 'it will finally succeed in rendering nuclear energy harmless'.

The experiment had been too dangerous to repeat with the limited facilities available; Reich realised that he must first find other ways of demonstrating orgone's usefulness. But at this point the US Food and Drug Administration intervened, securing an injunction against him in terms which it is hard to believe could have been proposed by such a body, let alone accepted by the courts. It represented, in effect, a sentence of death for orgone: 'All accumulators to be disassembled, all printed matter regarding orgone energy to be destroyed, on the ground that orgone energy does not exist.'

Understandably, but in the event unwisely, Reich maintained that what is or is not scientifically valid cannot be left to the courts; or, for that matter, the government, for this would be to make the government 'the final authority on matters of scientific research'. He began to try out orgone as a way of rain-making. First reports were encouraging; but the research was interrupted by the police. Charged with contempt of court for flouting the injunction, Reich was found guilty and sentenced to two years' imprisonment; and a heavy fine was levied on his institute. When his appeal failed, all his books and papers were incinerated; and he died in prison – according to his friends, of the Oranur sickness.

Describing the FDA's action in *The Pattern of Health*, Aubrey Westlake observed that it is hard to credit that this is a 'contemporary event'. There seems no good reason to doubt that something significant had happened, particularly as three weeks later, the *New York Times* reported an unexplained increase in radiation levels in a six hundred mile area around Oranur. Doubtless there might have been another explanation, but this could have been established by enquiry. If there was even a modicum of justification for Reich's theory, and of orgone's effect on radiation, it could have had extremely important consequences for medicine: pointing as it did to the possibility that radiation sickness was not, as was assumed, the direct consequence of nuclear radiations, but a symptom of the body's reaction, or over-reaction, to the radiation dose (Westlake cited the parallel of abscess formation, which could easily be mistaken for the work of the invading bacteria, but which in reality is the way the body's defence system manages to round them up, and contain them).

Had the FDA proceeded against Reich for conducting experiments which were a danger to the public it would have had every justification, to judge from Reich's own account of what happened. But this would have compelled admission of the possibility that Reich had discovered a hitherto unknown source of energy. The obvious alternative would have been to charge him with false pretences; but this would have given him the opportunity to try to prove, with the help of his gadgetry, that there was no pretence. So the FDA had chosen to crush him by a legal device from which there would be no escape. 'The haters of truth are still as powerful, if not more so, than they ever were,' Westlake concluded, 'and Reich, for all his genius, was overwhelmed.'

Reich was not the only victim of the sustained campaign against medical heterodoxy. Following Abrams' death, Ruth Drown had become the leading 'black box' practitioner in the United States, with her box designed on the 'rubbing-board oracle' principle, and with a new gadget, a 'camera'. If film were placed in it, it sometimes produced a picture of human organs not unlike an X-ray photograph, as if the symptoms had managed to insinuate themselves on to the negative; yet there was no exposure in the usual sense, as the 'camera' had no lens or shutter. This, if anything, made Drown even more hateful in orthodox eyes. When in 1950 she was persuaded to allow herself and her gadgets to be tested at the University of Chicago, the results were destructive of her reputation. 'Box' and 'Camera' produced wildly inaccurate diagnoses. In 1951 she was prosecuted, convicted and imprisoned; her instruments were impounded and destroyed; and soon after her release she died.

The best-known Brititsh radionics' practitioner, George de la Warr, also had to face legal action; but it was a civil case, and it had for him a happier outcome. De la Warr, who had a scientific training, clung to the belief that he could convince his fellow scientists of the objective reality of radionics as demonstrated by his devices, the 'box' and the 'camera'. What de la Warr could not bring himself to admit was that 'box' and 'camera', like pendulum or hazel twig, only gave convincing results when operated by particular individuals, and not always even then. When de la Warr sold his devices, therefore, some purchasers were unable to obtain any reaction; and in 1960 one of them sued him. De la Warr was lucky. The judge in the case, though sceptical, emphasised to the jury that they were not being asked to express an opinion about the scientific merits of de la Warr's contraptions; their function was simply to decide whether de la Warr was guilty of false pretences. If they felt he honestly believed in his method, they should find in his favour. They did.

SIDE-EFFECTS

On balance, unorthodox medicine had a hard time of it in the 1950s, with public opinion still bowled over by the triumphs of the wonder drugs. But one branch made a recovery; and this was largely because treatment with a new drug had unexpected and unwelcome consequences. What with surgery for slipped discs and cortisone for rheumatoid arthritis, osteopaths in Britain had been threatened with the defection of their patients; but slipped disc operations were so often useless (and sometimes disastrous) that they were ceasing to be fashionable, and cortisone's ugly limitations were quickly exposed. It removed symptoms as if by magic, but only temporarily; if taken for more than a few days its effects could be unpleasant (rashes, itches), unsightly (men became moonfaced, women hirsute), and sometimes terrifying (bouts of manic depression). It also impaired the body's defences against infection, encouraging the depradations of bacteria, and of viruses immune to antibiotics. And although cortisone was quickly replaced by its steroid derivatives, promoted as being free from its disadvantages, they were soon being indicted for many of the same side-effects. Before the end of the 1950s osteopathy was again in demand.

For a time, though, it was possible for the medical profession to think of cortisone as an unlucky exception to the general rule of sustained progress through the introduction of new drugs; particularly when, in 1955, the introduction of the Salk vaccine against polio seemed to confirm that medical science could continue to win spectacular victories in the war against disease. It had been hard enough for a Christian Scientist, let alone anybody who preferred homeopathy or herbal treatment, to resist the temptation to go to the doctor to obtain a prescription for an antibiotic, knowing that it could clear up their symptoms in a few hours. But it was far harder for parents to refuse to allow their children to be immunised against polio, knowing what friends and neighbours would say should their children catch the disease; knowing, too, that nobody would blame them if one of their children sickened and died as a consequence of the immunisation procedure.

Gradually, though, it was coming to be realised that all the wonder drugs, and not just cortisone, had drawbacks. Meyler's *Side Effects of Drugs*, published in 1952, showed that the range of adverse reactions was far more extensive than had been admitted. But by this time the pharmaceutical industry was immensely powerful: one of the most profitable industries in the world. And it had the backing of the medical profession, because doctors did not care to be told what drugs they could or could not use. Such side-effects, the public was assured, were a small price to pay for the benefits of the new drugs. How beneficial they had been was assiduously reiterated in the manufacturer's promotion, and rarely questioned in medical journals, most of them dependent for the bulk of their income from drug advertising. 'Thanks to antibiotics,' the *Journal of Antibiotic Medicine and Clinical Therapy* claimed in 1956, 'a million and a half lives were saved in the first fifteen years of the sulphonamide and antibiotic era.'

STRESS

Was this really true? Gale E. Wilson, a county doctor in Washington, had been afforded a curious opportunity to find out. As a County Coroner he was notified of all deaths which occurred when no medical attendant had been called in. Over a period of twenty years, therefore, he had examined, and where necessary autopsied, the bodies of over a thousand Christian Scientists. And by comparing the average age at which they died with the figures for the rest of the population, Wilson realised, he would be able to show the extent to which Christian Scientists had suffered because of their rejection of drug therapy.

The results, presented at the annual meeting of the American Academy of Forensic Sciences in 1956, were disconcerting. On balance, assuming the sample to be representative, Christian Scientists lived longer than the rest of the population. The only fault Wilson could find with them was that they were more prone to die of cancer than the rest of the population: they could have lived longer still, he argued, had they not been inclined to reject surgery. But, as the evidence has since revealed, surgery had not then substantially improved the chances of survival in the commoner forms of cancer. What was more significant, though Wilson did not realise it, was that for the two types of disease from which more Christian Scientists died than the rest of the population, cancer and heart attacks, there was no effective drug treatment. If any lesson was to be drawn from the comparison, antibiotics had not increased longevity; they had slightly diminished it.

Why? One possibility was put forward later that year in Hans Selye's *The Stress of Life*. Selye, Director of the Institute of Experimental Medicine in McGill University, Montreal, had found that if forcibly-immobilised laboratory rats were given a dose of irritant which ordinary had little or no effect on them, they would die. 'A rat wants to have his own way,' Selye reasoned, 'just like a human being.' Their frustration at being unable to move could be paralleled by human frustration in, say, a constricting job or an unhappy marriage. In such circumstances what made rats or people ill was not necessarily a virus or poison, but stress; not directly, but because it blew a fuse, as it were, in the body's homeostat. A few members of the medical profession welcomed Selye's theory, among them the surgeon Sir Heneage Ogilvie of Guy's Hospital, editor of *The Practitioner*. Ogilvie had advanced the proposition 'the happy man never gets cancer', admitting that he could not provide statistical proof but claiming that he had endlessly observed that its onset followed upon some disaster, a bereavement or an accident or a financial crisis, which suggested that the cause should be looked for not in a virus, but in the breakdown of the body's self-regulating system; and he hailed Selye's work as 'perhaps the greatest contribution to scientific medicine in the present century'. And in 1957 Arthur Guirdham, a psychiatrist practising in Bath, presented what was in effect confirmatory historical evidence in *A Theory of Disease*, showing how stress influenced the types of illnesses to which not just individuals, but whole communities, were prone.

The medical Establishment, however, remained unimpressed. The stress theory, relating symptoms as it did to everyday conflicts, was rather less unpalatable than the psychosomatic theory, with its Freudian undertones; but specialists could not actively welcome it because it would spoil their search for *the* cause of whatever disease they specialised in: germ, or virus, or chemical or gene. They fell back on the argument that as people had had more stressful lives in earlier periods of history, owing to war, pestilence and famine, stress could not really be the culprit; thereby showing they had missed Selye's point, which was that it is the individual frustration arising out of constricted urban living, rather than life's major causes of worry, which make people illness-prone. And this failure to appreciate the implications of the stress theory, provoking as it did dissatisfaction with orthodoxy, led to what is often the first indication of such dissatisfaction; an increase in the number of articles, tracts and books examining the alternatives. In 1958 three substantial surveys appeared: Jean Palaiseul's massive four volume *Au-delà de la médécine: tous les moyens de vous guérir interdits aux médécins*; Heinz Graupner's *Wer Heilt hat Recht*; and Geoffrey Murray's *Frontiers of Healing*.

Of these, Palaiseul's account of various healing methods practised in Europe, often in spite of rigorous laws against unqualified practitioners, was the most detailed. It revealed the range of treatments which were available – at least for anybody who took the trouble to search them out; and usually it took trouble, as most of them were unfamiliar. A few un-orthodox methods had established themselves all over the Western world: osteopathy, chiropractic, homeopathy, nature cure, herbalism. Some others had survived, precariously, in a few centres: Priessnitz's and Kneipp's water cure and Coué's auto-suggestion still had their devotees. Some had surfaced because they had been in the news: as Professor Niehans' cellular therapy had reputedly just saved the life of Pope Pius XII, it had been widely written up in the popular press. Most were, and were to remain, obscure.

Palaiseul did not deal with spiritual or psychic healing; but Murray included Christian Science, Lourdes and radiesthesia, along with osteopathy. Graupner was chiefly concerned with remedies from 'nature's medicine chest', some rendered respectable, like the moulds from which antibiotics were obtained; some still suspect, like injections of 'royal jelly' from beehives. But between the three of them the authors had provided the first introduction to what for the great majority of their readers must have been almost unknown territory. They showed that although unqualified practitioners had survived, only a few of them could be said to flourish. Occasionally an osteopath or a healer might build up a fashionable practice, as Barker had done; but the great majority attracted public notice only if they were prosecuted for breaking some law. Organisationally, too, they were in no condition to cope with any increase in demand for their services. Even where they had managed to form national bodies, splits had occurred which reduced their effectiveness, and left them with no prospect of winning the confidence either of the public or of legislators.

Chapter Six

EAST MEETS WEST

Recalling the doctrines of Helmont and Paracalsus at the 1959 psycho-analyst congress in Copenhagen, Marie Bonaparte suggested that what medicine in the 1950s had been witnessing – renewed interest in the mind and the emotions – was nothing less than a revival of vitalism. The term by that time had slipped sufficiently far out of colloquial usage for most doctors to regard it as archaic rather than sinister. Vitalism was long since dead; nothing, surely, could bring it back to life! The assumption remained that there was nothing for orthodoxy to worry about which medical science in general, and the pharmaceutical industry in particular, could not set right.

Nevertheless warnings continued to be given from time to time; and not just by rebels or mavericks. René Dubos was a bacteriologist – he had discovered one of the antibiotics – and a disciple of Pasteur, whose biography he had written. But he was disturbed by the mounting toll of side-effects; by the development of strains of pathogenic bacteria resistant to antibiotics; and by the signs that the public was becoming dangerously drug-dependent. People must realise, he pleaded in his *Mirage of Health,* published in 1959, that advances in medical technology could not bring good health. 'Is it not an illusion,' he asked, 'to proclaim the present state of health as the best in the history of the world, at a time when increasing numbers of persons in our society depend on drugs and doctors for meeting the ordinary problems of everyday life?'

There were other indications of growing dissatisfaction with mechanism in the medical profession. A. T. W. Simeons' *Man's Presumptuous Brain,* a study of the evolutionary process which explained much of what had been obscure about the genesis of psychosomatic and stress disorders; and Ronald Laing's *The Divided Self,* with its plea that psychosis should be regarded not as a breakdown but, at least potentially, as a breakthrough. Laing was later to become a cult figure, but at the time it was the work of another doctor which made the biggest impression. D. C. Jarvis's *Folk Medicine* was a plea for a return to natural remedies, based on his observations of animal life in the course of his work as a general practitioner in Vermont.

Animals, Jarvis reminded his readers, 'know unerringly which herb will cure what ills'. An animal with fever would rest near water, drinking plenty of it but eating nothing until it is recovered. 'On the other hand, an animal bedevilled by rheumatism finds a spot of hot sunlight and lies in it until the misery bakes out.' Although it was over-simplified – as was his stock prescription; two teaspoonfuls of honey and two teaspoonfuls of apple-cider vinegar in a glass of water every day – Jarvis's theme caught the public fancy. The book stayed in *Time*'s list of the top ten best sellers for over a year, suggesting the possibility that there could be a keen demand for natural medicine in the United States, if it were better understood and more readily available.

THALIDOMIDE

Soon the demand was to make itself felt: not as a result of any propaganda for unorthodox methods, but from an episode which revealed orthodoxy's limitations.

In the summer of 1961 a report was published of the findings of a committee set up in America under Senator Kefauver to investigate price fixing in the pharmaceutical industry. The evidence showed that a number of companies, including some of the largest, had not merely rigged prices: they had lied to the medical profession about the safety of their products, in some cases continuing to promote them as safe even after their own medical advisers had warned them that dangerous side-effects were being reported. The attitude of the medical profession in Britain, as reflected in the medical journals, was complacent: 'it could not happen here'. But in fact similar warnings had been given, and were being given, to the Distillers' Company in Britain, whose pharmaceutical branch had marketed a sedative, thalidomide, with the trade name Distaval. Effective though the drug undoubtedly was it had been associated with side-effects of a kind which were sufficiently disturbing to convince Dr Frances Kelsey, of the Food and Drug Administration in Washington, that it should not be granted a licence in the United States until more exhaustively tested – much to the indignation of Merrell and Co. who were to market it there.

Distillers ignored the warnings. Even when an article appeared in the *British Medical Journal* in the autumn of 1961, describing how patients treated with thalidomide in a London hospital had developed peripheral neuropathy – numbness in the fingers and toes, impairment of sensation and other symptoms, some of which 'resembled neuropathy associated with malignant disease', and which did not disappear when the treatment with the drug was discontinued – the Distillers' Company not merely refused to withdraw the drug (a decision supported by an editorial in the *BMJ*) but continued to promote it, emphasising in their advertisements how safe it was (which the *BMJ* continued to accept). Only when, in November, reports from Germany showed that thalidomide had been associated with birth deformities was the drug at last withdrawn.

There was no immediate scandal. It was not for some months, in fact, that any British newspaper had the courage to tell the story, for fear of the Distillers' Company lawyers. But when the public began to grasp what had happened, confidence in drugs, and to a lesser extent in the doctors, was shaken. Thalidomide was exceptional, as an investigation into other drug scandals by an American Senate Committee under Hubert Humphrey was to reveal, only because of the children's deformities – much as a quarter of a century earlier, polio had become the most dreaded of diseases because victims were so often identifiable for life. The impact in the United States was not so great: fewer than twenty thalidomide children were born there (as against an estimated ten thousand had the FDA allowed it to be marketed). But in other countries the thalidomide children – about six thousand, of them in West Germany alone – periodically reminded the public, when they appeared in the news or on television programmes, of the hazards of treatment by powerful new drugs, and of the failure of the medical profession to exercise adequate control over their marketing.

ACUPUNCTURE

The outcome of the affair was an immediate upsurge of interest in unorthodox medical theories and practices; and the first beneficiary was acupuncture.

When and how acupuncture originated remains a mystery, but it seems likely that it developed out of a practice observed in tribal communities where sickness was treated by scarification of the skin, to let out blood or pus, or evil substances. Flints, or thorns, were used, and sometimes the shaman would invest them with psychic significance by conjuring them up to his aid. In his *Fleurs Noirs et Ames Blanches* Fr Trilles, recalling experience as a missionary in French Equatorial Africa around the end of the nineteenth century, described an episode in which he was invited to watch a witch-doctor provide treatment. As nobody else was in the vicinity Trilles had been astonished to observe 'numbers of small, fine needles, white and sharp' appearing on the patient's body, particularly round the part where pain had been felt, piercing the flesh to about a millimetre. Examining them, Trilles found they were long white thorns. He could think of no explanation. Black Africa, he had to admit, 'had its secrets, of which old Europe is unaware'.

Old Europe was not wholly unaware of the psychic significance of small sharp objects, commonly reported as materialising in cases of demonic possession and witchcraft. Needles were also used by doctors in what they described as acupuncture to release fluid in cases of dropsy; one such case was related in the first issue of the *Lancet* in 1823 by Dr John Tweedale, from King's Lynn in Norfolk. 'For lumbago,' Osler wrote in the 1912 edition of his *Principles and Practice of Medicine,* 'acupuncture is in acute cases the most efficient treatment'; the method he used was to thrust needles into the lumbar muscles at the seat of pain, and withdraw them after five to ten minutes. But in the absence of any satisfactory explanation why the method worked, it had fallen into disuse, except in China and other far eastern countries, where it had become a standard therapeutic technique.

Chinese acupuncture was more sophisticated than the Western variety. The earliest surviving manuals, dating from around five thousand years ago, show that the needles were already being inserted at specific points, depending on the outcome of the diagnosis; and that the diagnosis itself was being obtained with the help of pulse-taking, the 'feel' of the pulse, as well as its regularity, rate and vigour, being taken into consideration. The theory was that the life force functions through the flow of energy through certain channels; and if there is a blockage, illness results. The needles were used to stimulate the energy flow through the appropriate channel, until equilibrium was restored.

Acupuncture continued to be standard practice in China and some other eastern countries; but apart from France, where it became fairly familiar owing to the impression it had made on colonial officials, missionaries and traders in French colonies, the eastern version had hardly been heard of in the West except in Chinatowns in maritime cities. The editor of a London women's magazine which published an article on it as a curiosity in 1960 was consequently staggered when ten thousand letters poured in, most of them from people who wanted to know where they could get the treatment. There were a handful of doctors who practised it in Britain; one of them, Felix Mann, had written a book on the subject, and he was inundated with requests for treatment. Mann realised the need for more practitioners; but he held the view that like himself they must be medically qualified, and this would have restricted the number which could be recruited even if the attitude in the profession to the new craze had not been openly contemptuous. Although Mann hoped to be able to show that, as he believed, acupuncture had a straightforward basis in physiology ('the nerve fibres of the automatic nervous system are stimulated') the idea was ridiculed by neurologists, who pointed out that the acupuncture points and models bore no relation to the channels of the automatic nervous system.

Inevitably practitioners who were not medically qualified presented themselves to fill the gap. Anybody who had acquired a smattering of the craft could practise it, at least under British law, and teach it to others; and within a couple of years acupuncture clinics were to be found in most of the larger cities. The medical journals periodically fulminated against them; but acupuncturists could do little harm unless they failed to sterilise their needles. The profession's chief argument against them, too – that they might deter patients from seeking proper treatment – was irrelevant. The vast majority of people who tried acupuncture had tried the 'proper' treatment, and found it wanting.

Another common criticism was that acupuncturists attracted most of their custom from people with disorders such as rheumatoid arthritis and backache, which were subject to remissions anyway, and even if the remission were not coincidental, it could have been induced through suggestion. The criticism would have had more force if the doctors themselves had not been exploiting suggestion, while pretending to patients (and often to themselves) that it was the drug that was effective. There was to be a striking example of this in the 1960's, when indomethacin, marketed by Merck as Indocid (in the US, Indocin) was introduced as a new anti-inflammatory drug to replace the discredited steroids. Soon afterwards reports of trials in the *New England Journal of Medicine* and in the *British Medical Journal* showed that patients treated with aspirin, or even with a placebo, did as well as or better than those treated with indomethacin. The reports were ignored. Indomethacin was promoted to general practitioners in a massive campaign; GPs in turn assured patients it was wonderful; and for some patients it was. In all probability they would have done just as well on tablets of bicarbonate of soda or lactose; but their doctors were not going to tell them that.

Like the steroids, indomethacin had some unpleasant side-effects; and the growing public realisation that side-effects were an inexorable accompaniment of orthodox drug therapy began to divert patients from GP's surgeries to fringe practitioners. People who had suffered from the common steroid side-effects – rashes, dry mouth, headaches, general malaise – had put up with them as the price they had to pay to escape pain, but the thalidomide affair and later scandals set them wondering whether the price in the form of long-term risk might not be too high. Partly through a spate of articles on the various unorthodox methods in popular magazines, partly through word of mouth, medically unqualified practitioners who had formerly worked in obscurity now found themselves sought out. Their organisations, which had been hard put to it to survive the lean years, began to recover and to attract new recruits.

HERBALISM

The herbalists, in particular, were quick to realise the opportunity they had been afforded by the public's worry about synthetic drugs. Inevitably herbalism had been the branch of natural medicine which had suffered most at the hands of medical science. Since the early years of the nineteenth century it had come to be accepted that if certain plants had yet to yield up their healing secrets, as the foxglove and Peruvian bark had done, it would not be the plant itself that would be used, but some extract, 'refined' and 'purified' to convert it into a chemical which could then be tested, weighed, packaged and sold across a chemist's counter, thereby ensuring profit for the manufacturer and the chemist, and the security of a well-regulated product for the doctor and his patients. The lure of profit understandably also induced herbalists of talent to move into the refining and packaging area. Two of the greatest names in the history of patent medicines had begun as herbalists. Thomas Beecham – father of the conductor – won a local reputation for his knowledge of herbs while working as a shepherd boy; his pills and powders were to make him a millionaire. Jesse Boot's father ran a herbalist's shop; Jesse studied pharmacy, opened first one and then a chain of chemist's shops, and by 1910 had built up the world's biggest pharmaceutical retail group.

Edward Bach moved in the reverse direction. Before the

First World War he had established himself as a bacteriologist with a successful London practice; but in the 1920's his
researches convinced him of the value of homeopathic treatment. From this he moved on to study herbalism; and in the
last years of his life – he died in 1936 – he revived theories
and practices which reached far back into the past. Bach believed in intuition as a guide to the discovery of the right
plant medicines – much as tribal medicine men had, and as
witches did in folklore. He believed, too, that the therapeutic
effect of herbs did not depend simply on the chemicals they
contained; they could 'draw down spiritual power, which
cleanses mind and body and heals'. He was not just advocat-
ing a revival of Culpeper-style herbalism; implicit in his thesis
were links with homeopathy, radiesthesia and healing. But in
this he was in advance of his time. Although disciples continued his work, most herbalists had repudiated him as at best
a visionary, at worst the victim of occult superstitions which
could only bring their cause into disrepute.

Whether they were attracted by Bach's ideas, or irritated by
them, herbalists in the early 1960's felt they could say 'we
told you so!' with every justification. In her *Green Medicine*,
published in 1950 at the height of cortisone's initial fame,
Hilda Leyel had pointed out its link with the plant from
which African natives extracted poison to put on the tips of
their arrows. If used medicinally, she advised, it should be
given as a tincture of the whole plant, 'because the therapeutic derivatives are the poisonous parts of the plant, and
contain none of the foods which are found in the natural
state'; a reiteration of the traditional argument that herbal
remedies were designed by nature to be taken as a whole, the
various ingredients complementing each other, and providing
safeguards which were lost if the particular chemicals were 'refined', and extracted from the rest.

In the early 1960's, encouraged by the number of enquiries
from people worried about drugs, the National Institute of
Medical Herbalists in Britain set up an ambitious training
scheme, offering students a five-year course including biology,
physiology, and allied subjects, which would have put them on
a par with the osteopaths, as they would be turning out fifty

qualified herbalists a year. It proved to be a false dawn. Fifty students were duly enrolled, but many found the training wearisome. They had had visions of themselves, perhaps, gathering and preparing herbal remedies, rather than as students listening to boring lectures on the human body. Many dropped out, and the following year only five newcomers enrolled. Other fringe groups had similar, though less serious, setbacks. The osteopaths in Britain had prepared for a massive expansion. It, too, did not materialise.

There were various reasons for the inability of the unorthodox practices to establish themselves, but the main one was that orthodox medicine was in too commanding a position. Although the Ministry of Health might battle with the British Medical Association over pay and status, few governments were prepared to intervene in what they regarded as medical affairs. When Enoch Powell as Minister tried to break the pharmaceutical industry's international cartel by cutting down on some patents – a justifiable retaliation, as some of the biggest companies in the United States had obtained their antibiotic patents by false pretences, and were convicted of price-rigging as a consequence – he found that the industry was supported by the medical profession; and his Labour successor, Kenneth Robinson, feebly gave way to their combined pressure. The industry by this time had immense reserves at its disposal; and it was able to ladle out reassurance. There could be no more thalidomide disasters, it claimed, because a Government-backed committee had been set up to ensure that all new drugs were suitably tested before being marketed. The industry, having learned from its errors, was poised for fresh advances.

It was; thanks to *Rauwolfia serpentina*, or snake-root. It had been used from time immemorial in India as a mild relaxant (it was favoured by Gandhi as a nightcap); and in 1949 an article in the *British Heart Journal* disclosed that after ten years of trials there, it had been found also to be effective in the treatment of high blood pressure. Trials at the Massachusetts General Hospital confirmed that the snake-root preparations used were not just another addition to the then rapidly growing list of heart drugs; they had also shown encouraging results in the treatment of tension, so they might help in dealing with neuroses. The result was that reserpine, regarded as the root's main constituent, was isolated, and eventually synthesised: the drug, the first of the tranquillisers, enjoyed enormous sales; and by the 1960s its successors were giving their manufacturers higher profits than ever.

Orthodoxy, therefore, was recovering its temporarily-shaken confidence; and although Morton Mintz's *The Therapeutic Nightmare*, a well-documented survey published in 1965 of the Kefauver hearings and the subsequent sparring between the FDA, the medical profession and the pharmaceutical industry, appeared damning ('I read it,' John Kenneth Galbraith commented, 'with horror and fascination'), it had no lasting effect. Whenever proposals were put forward to improve the safety or reduce the price of drugs, the drug companies would warn the doctors that this would be the thin edge of the socialised medicine wedge; and between them the industry and the profession could muster so powerful a lobby in Washington that they could prevent, or at least emasculate, projected reforms.

AUTOGENIC TRAINING: BIOFEEDBACK

Forces were at work, though, away from the political arena which were beginning to undermine the premises of orthodox medicine: and the first indication that the threat might be serious, like the sudden collapse of floor boards revealing dry rot, was a quick succession of events in 1969, an *annus mirabilis* for all those struggling to free medicine from mechanist domination.

One was the publication of a report from Neal E. Miller, Professor of Physiological Psychology at Rockefeller University in New York. Laboratory rats, he claimed, could learn how to increase or decrease their heart rates. They could even control the flow of blood to their ears, raising it or lowering the ear temperature. It had been known for years that by rewards and punishments, cheese or electric shocks, rats could be taught to go the correct way through a maze, to lift hatches or to open doors, and to perform other similar feats. But

Miller's rats had displayed the ability to meddle with the workings of their autonomic nervous systems, normally regarded as self-governing.

And if rats could do it, why not people? As it happened, some experiments had already begun. In 1968 a group of students became interested in the type of yoga, Transcendental Meditation, which had been introduced to the West by the Maharishi. They came to Herbert Benson, Associate Professor of Medicine at the Harvard Medical School, saying that they believed they could use TM to lower their blood pressure. In *The Relaxation Response* Benson has recalled that as the staff were busy at the time studying the blood pressure of monkeys, the students were turned away. 'Why investigate anything so far out as meditation?' But the students persisted; and eventually Benson was persuaded that what they proposed was worth trying. The experiment was conducted on traditional behaviourist lines: the meditators' blood pressure was monitored, and if they succeeded in lowering it they were rewarded with a look at a picture of a *Playboy* nude. Whether or not the inducement was needed the method worked; and the outcome was the remarkable spectacle of Benson, the behaviourist, eulogising the techniques of the yogi, whose claims behaviourists had so long and often so pointedly ignored.

That the mind could exercise some control of this kind was not in fact a new discovery. In his lectures on surgery, delivered in 1786–7, John Hunter described how he had been to a 'magnetiser' not because he believed in animal magnetism but because he wanted to try out a theory he had formulated: that any part of the body could be influenced by the imagination if it were 'worked up by attention to the part expected to be affected'. When the magnetiser told him that he would have a feeling in his hand, he concentrated instead on his big toe, and duly had the feeling there. 'I am confident,' he concluded, 'that I can fix my attention to any part until I have a sensation in that part.' Braid, too, experimenting with some of his hypnotised subjects in the 1840's, found that if he told them to concentrate on the palms of their hands for a few minutes they would report altered sensations of various kinds: cold, warmth or pins-and-needles. And around the time Coué's auto-suggestion was becoming internationally celebrated, the German doctor Johannes Schultz had initiated a similar method. Like Coué, he had adapted it from the work of earlier investigators of hypnotism, who had found that some of their subjects were able to learn to put themselves into the trance state; they could then save time and trouble by doing for themselves what the hypnotist had been doing for them. Also like Coué, Schultz came to realise that hypnotism was unnecessary: a course of 'autogenic training', as he called it, would enable patients to do all that was necessary for themselves. And among the lessons was one in which they trained themselves to influence their blood circulation. By reciting to themselves 'my hands are warm,' they could make their hands warm.

Although Schultz himself commanded respect among his colleagues, his work had not made any perceptible impact within the medical profession. The comfortable assumption had continued to be that the autonomic nervous system was self-governing. Admittedly it responded to a variety of emotional stimuli. But this automatic response to stimuli was the function of the system; an indication that the homeostatic mechanism was operating efficiently. The individual could interfere by, say, removing himself from the stimuli. Somebody at the scene of an accident could leave, to avoid the effects of shock from seeing blood. But the idea that people could alter their own blood pressure had hardly been considered.

The implications of Miller's and Benson's research were far-reaching. By the 1960s high blood pressure had come to be regarded as, and treated as, a disease, even when there were no obvious symptoms, because it was known to be associated with an increased risk of heart attacks. The ability to lower it by meditation would consequently be extremely valuable, as being both cheaper and safer than lowering it by drugs. The problem was that except in a laboratory people had no means of knowing whether their blood pressure was being lowered. What was needed was some device like a thermometer, which would relay the required information back to the meditator.

One psycho-physiological monitoring device had already attracted a great deal of attention, and some notoriety. The principle on which it worked had been discovered by the French psychologist Charles Féré, one of Charcot's Salpêtrière group. Investigating animal magnetism with a view to finding some acceptable rational explanation, Féré had made experiments with magnets and electric currents, which showed that the resistance of the skin to a small amount of current altered with changes in the patient's mood. This had given Jung the idea of wiring up patients to a meter while they were taking his word-association tests, so that he could detect which words were loaded with an emotional charge. But for some reason – probably, Barbara Brown has suggested in her *New Mind, New Body*, because Pavlov's methods so fascinated the physiologically-orientated psychologists that they switched their attention from human beings to rats and monkeys, and the behaviourists had carried on the work – this clue was not followed up by the medical profession. The method was, however, used in connection with criminal investigations, with the help of 'lie-detectors' working on the same principle as Jung's gadget. Although they were not an entirely reliable guide, they did at least continue to show that alterations in an individual's emotional condition could be displayed by mechanical means: a technique which came to be identified with 'biofeedback'.

In a sense, the tribal diviner who employed a pendulum or a rubbing-board oracle to answer the questions he was putting to himself was using biofeedback. So was the radionic practitioner plucking at the rubber in his 'black box'. But orthodox medicine had dismissed such devices as occultist; and no steps were taken to develop biofeedback for therapeutic purposes until in the mid-1960s Elmer Green and his wife, impressed by the autogenic training course which they had taken at the Menninger Foundation in Texas, began themselves to teach it to students. They found that the students did better when they were able to observe their own progress, for example by obtaining visual evidence that they were increasing or decreasing the temperature in one hand before the change became perceptible in the ordinary way. Soon, biofeedback was also being used to convey information about changes in brain rhythms, offering the prospect of helping people to reduce tensions; and in 1969, one hundred and forty people interested in the subject came together for a three-day meeting at which The Biofeedback Research Society was formed.

Barbara Brown has recalled the exhilaration felt by the participants on that occasion. The medical Establishment could no longer deny that its resistance to psychosomatic and stress theories had been based on fallacious reasoning about the limitations of the mind's influence on the body. But it could do what it had done before, and claim that the discoveries of the researchers in the 1960s were of no clinical significance. One eminent American authority, according to Barbara Brown, told a conference that the fact that autonomic functions such as heart rate could be brought under control was probably of no importance whatsoever: 'All that it means is that we have a new way to continue our studies.' In Britain most doctors, hearing of autogenic training and biofeedback, dismissed them as only another fad. When they were demonstrated on television or described in the press they were ordinarily presented as unorthodox, even if being used by a member of the medical profession.

THE CHINESE DIMENSION

Nevertheless orthodoxy could not entirely disguise the fact it had suffered a setback; and worse was soon to follow. Autogenic training and biofeedback could at least be herded into psycho-physiological quarantine, along with stress and psychosomatics; treated as things which required more elucidation in scientific terms before they could be accepted. Acupuncture was a different matter. Not merely did it break the rules, it broke them in what for orthodoxy was a singularly humiliating fashion.

So manifestly absurd had acupuncture appeared that doctors ordinarily mentioned it only in derision. A typical example had been the reference to it by the American pharmacologist, Louis Lasagna, in his trenchant *The Doctors' Dilemmas*, published in 1962. Acupuncture featured in his chapter on 'Superstition and Ignorance' as one of his list of 'lunacies' (most of them, to do him justice, had been orthodox in their time:

bleeding, cupping, purging). The charts which had been drawn up to help the practitioner place his needles, Lasagna sarcastically suggested, had been necessary only because 'hitting imaginary canals is not a job to be left to the imagination'.

Then, in 1971, James Reston of the *New York Times* went down with appendicitis while he was on a visit to China; and following an operation he was given acupuncture ('three long needles inserted into the outer part of my right elbow and below my knees') to relieve him of stomach distension. As he reported in the *Times*, the treatment worked. The incident might have been forgotten, but Chairman Mao happened to be a zealous advocate of acupuncture (probably for political rather than for clinical reasons); and the Chinese Medical Association, either at his prompting or with his blessing, invited American doctors to see Chinese medicine for themselves, including the internationally-celebrated cardiologist, Paul Dudley White of Boston, E. Grey Dimond, Provost of the Health Sciences Department of the University of Missouri, and Professor Samuel Rosen, of the Mount Sinai School of Medicine. What they witnessed convinced them. They were particularly impressed by acupuncture anesthesia (strictly speaking, analgesia). The mesmerists had had to wait over a hundred years before their claim that surgery could be rendered painless was accepted by the profession, because the fact that mesmerised patients appeared to be asleep could be attributed to the fact that they were steeling themselves to bear the pain. But the patients in Chinese hospitals remained wide awake even during the most serious operations. 'It is an extraordinary experience,' Rosen reported, 'to see a patient lying relaxed and awake, sipping tea, on an operating table, an acupuncturist twirling a needle about two inches long above her wrist, while a tuberculous lung is being removed.'

It was hard to accept that three such experienced doctors had allowed themselves to be duped; and soon, visits to China by other teams of doctors from the United States and from Europe, as well as films of operations with acupuncture as the pain-killer, confirmed not merely that it worked, but that it worked extremely effectively. 'The scarcely-veiled thought that acupuncture is some kind of hoax has lifted',

Science (a journal which ordinarily made little attempt to veil its thoughts about such matters) had to admit, a year after Reston's dispatch had appeared; most Western scientists now agreed that 'acupuncture works'.

There could hardly have been a more devastating exposure of the limitations of western-style orthodox medicine. It was clear from the reports that few, if any, of the doctors who visited China to investigate acupuncture had even considered investigating it in their home towns. Most of them would not have crossed the road to see an acupuncturist at work; they would have felt it improper to countenance such quackery. And if they had investigated acupuncture and found that it worked, in all probability they would have kept quiet about it, to avoid the ridicule of their colleagues. Now, disconcertingly, they were confronted with the fact that the unbelievable had to be believed; and they had to decide what to do about it.

Predictably, the first reaction was to claim that for the safety of the community acupuncture should be taken over by the medical profession. 'We've got to get ahead of the fad that's surely going to develop,' Dimond insisted; otherwise, charlatans would move in to take advantage of 'a vast number of human pin-cushions'. It obviously had not occurred to Dimond that members of a profession which had refused even to investigate acupuncture, and had been treating it as a joke, were not necessarily the most suitable people to practise it. And even if they had been suitable, there were so few medically qualified acupuncturists – most of whom were soon overwhelmed with lucrative work, as a result of the publicity – that acupuncture could never be made generally available unless provision were made for the training of the equivalent of China's 'barefoot doctors'. And any such notion would certainly be strenuously resisted by the medical Establishments in America and Europe; supported by the pharmaceutical industry, which had nothing to gain from acupuncture's spread.

Chapter Seven

VITALISM REVISITED

In the light of history the medical profession could have been expected to make a quick recovery from the embarrassment of having to tolerate auto-suggestion, biofeedback and acupuncture. They could be treated as gate-crashers who could not be ejected but who might be contained, as mesmerism had eventually been contained. There was always the excuse to fall back on that more research would be needed before they could be given formal accreditation; whether the research was carried out would then depend on the money available, and it was safe to assume it would not be plentiful, as the pharmaceutical industry would not be enthusiastic contributors.

By the 1970s, however, the social scene was changing in ways which were beginning to have an effect on the public's attitudes to medicine. As Barbara Brown observed, biofeedback appeared during the period of social upheaval in the late 1960s, and may have contributed to it. University students, in particular, were challenging accepted beliefs and customs, preferring marihuana to alcohol, using LSD to try to open the doors of perception, 'exploring inner space'. The jargon might often be excruciating – 'psychobabble', as R. D. Rosen christened it, blocking rather than letting in the light; but the desire for illumination was real.

Unorthodox medical practices had formerly appealed chiefly to the elderly. The waiting rooms of herbalists and osteopaths had been filled with people who had exhausted orthodox medicine's resources, and were awaiting their turn not because they believed in the treatment they were about to receive but because they were desperate, willing to try anything. By the mid-1970s this had changed: the elderly were still there, but they had been joined by people in their twenties, or younger, who had rejected orthodox ideas, or had been caught up in one of the Eastern cults which had begun to take root in the West. And they were not likely to return to their former doctors until orthodox medicine came up with something new, to justify itself.

MEDICAL NEMESIS

Orthodoxy, however, was on its own evaluation beginning to slide. In surgery the ecstatic welcome for the first heart transplant in 1968 quickly gave way to disillusionment, which not even the more cautious and relatively successful operations at the Stanford University Medical Centre have dispelled. For a time the 'beta-blockers' were hailed as a breakthrough in the treatment of high blood pressure; but it would have been wiser for the medical profession to heed the warning given by William Evans a few years earlier when he recalled that he had seen over fifty such remedies marketed; that the earlier ones, though harmless, were useless; that the later ones, though more potent, had distressing side-effects; and that as drugs did not affect the cause of high blood pressure they should be discontinued. The beta-blockers were lavishly promoted and enthusiastically prescribed until one of them, Eraldin, was found to have such ugly side-effects, including blindness, that it had to be withdrawn; and the value of the others has yet to be proved.

The side-effects of drugs were to be the main ground for the fierce attack mounted by Ivan Illich in his *Medical Nemesis,* published in 1975. 'The Medical Establishment has become a major threat to health,' he claimed in his introduction: 'The disabling impact of professional control over medicine has reached the proportions of an epidemic' – a case which he proceeded to document with a wealth of evidence taken from medical journals. And although Illich's cantankerous style often alienated doctors who were sympathetic to his theme, there were many signs of increasing willingness within the profession to accept that reform was needed. But the existence of a self-perpetuating oligarchy controlling entry, training, qualifications and promotion proved a barrier to any but the most gradual change.

Even if the will were there, too, it would take many years to transform medical training; and in the meantime doctors would find it hard to change their attitudes and habits. 'The emotionally blunting effect of brainwashing during an allopathic training has to be experienced to be believed,' Alec Forbes – an NHS consultant practising in Plymouth – recalled in his *Try Being Healthy*, published in 1976. 'It takes many years to recover from it. Most of its products never do.'

Forbes was one of a group who had come together to form 'The Scientific and Medical Network', designed to challenge accepted orthodox assumptions; and as some of them feared that their prospects might be jeopardised if their defection to the enemy (as colleagues might regard it) became known, its membership list was kept secret until the Network's existence was discovered and described by a medical journalist, Robert Eagle, in the *Observer*. But by this time there was the first indication of a change of heart in the General Medical Council. In *Try Being Healthy* Forbes advocated that some unorthodox practitioners should be absorbed into the National Health Service; and this was obviously incompatible with the GMC's century-old ruling that any doctor who co-operated with a medically unqualified practitioner could be struck off the Register. But a few months later the GMC quietly and without fuss altered its rule. In future a doctor would be allowed to send patients to practitioners of any kind, provided that he had satisfied himself that they were equipped to treat the cases he referred to them, and so long as he retained the ultimate responsibility for each case.

Such was the suspicion which the actions of the GMC had aroused in the past that some paramedical practitioners suspected a trick. The plan, they suggested, was to make it more, not less, risky for a doctor to send patients to them. In the past he could simply have made it clear to patients that if they decided to go to an osteopath or a healer, he did not want to be told. He would then have had the simple defence, if brought up before the GMC, that he had not known. Now, he would be expected to exercise his discretion. He would know that so long as he continued to send patients to the consultants at the local hospital, even if he thought their methods useless or dangerous, nobody could blame him for their mistakes. But if mistakes were made by medically-unqualified practitioners to whom he had referred them, he could be in trouble.

The suspicion has proved to be unjustified. Although it has taken time for doctors to throw off old habits, and to learn to trust alternative practitioners, the advantage to the GP of the relaxation of the old rule outweighs the risks. Every GP has in his practice a proportion of patients whom he is compelled to see from time to time, though he knows there is little he can do for them except prescribe tranquillisers and pain killers. As Lord Winstanley – himself a GP – has hinted in a parliamentary debate, they are coming to realise what a relief it can be if patients take their chronic backaches to an osteopath, or their rheumatism to an acupuncturist.

In a document prepared for submission to the Royal Commission set up to investigate the National Health Service, the Healing Research Trust (of which Forbes is chairman) lists eight natural therapies which could come within the N.H.S.'s scope: acupuncture, chiropractic, herbalism, homeopathy, naturopathy, osteopathy, radionics and healing. There is one obvious, and striking, omission: psychotherapy. The difficulty here is partly that so many of the unorthodox varieties of psychotherapy available are provided by doctors or clinical psychologists and partly that it is not easy to decide whether certain mind-orientated cults or sects ought to be regarded as essentially religious rather than therapeutic. For the present, though, the eight named by the Healing Research Trust are those which are in line for recognition.

In the past, the main argument against the acceptance of such unorthodox practices has been that their value was unproven. This is now one of the least of their representatives' worries. The chief reason why their value was unproven was simply that the medical Establishment would not accept as valid the results of any research project unless they had themselves been involved in it; but with very rare exceptions, such as the Horder investigation of the radionic 'black box' in 1924, they had refused to allow themselves to become involved. Recently, however, a fair amount of research has been done, some of it by medical scientists, into all eight – or nine, including psychotherapy; and with some interesting results.

NATUROPATHY

Of all the forms of traditional medicine naturopathy has for years been taken the least seriously – except in Germany, and there it is more closely identified with orthodox medicine. In Britain it has usually conjured up a picture of large country houses set in parkland where well-off businessmen and their wives arrive periodically, (and often separately) for a week or two to 'dry out' and lose weight on a diet of lettuce and lemon juice. When Stanley Lief opened 'Champney's', in Hertfordshire, in the 1920's, he followed the Kneipp model, emphasising the desirability of outdoor exercise, lying in the sun (when there was sun) and rolling in the snow (when there was snow); but he was chiefly concerned with the provision of a healthful diet. This ought to have kept down prices but supernumerary therapies began to insinuate themselves in such establishments: massage, manipulation, electrical treatments, along with swimming pools, tennis courts, golf courses and, inevitably, television sets, so that by the 1970s it cost more to stay in some of them than it did to stay in country hotels of a similar character, with full board.

Many, probably most, of the people who patronise such establishments do so as a kind of penance for over-indulgence, well aware that the moment they leave they will resume their former eating, drinking and smoking habits. In more austere establishments, though, like the London Nature Cure Clinic, it is assumed that people who attend are genuinely seeking instruction on how to lead healthier lives. The recommended diet is strictly vegetarian, but it is not spartan; anybody who acquires a taste for vegetarian food would have no difficulty in maintaining it.

Like most nature cure establishments the clinic makes provision for homeopathic and osteopathic treatment, as well as various forms of hydrotherapy; but the naturopaths insist that their primary objective is prevention. And medical research in the past few years has been confirming their claims, particularly in connection with heart disease. In almost all affluent communities in all parts of the world, epidemiologists have found that certain 'risk factors' are associated with the onset of heart attacks, among them heavy smoking, excessive consumption of animal fats, inadequate exercise and obesity – the very culprits naturopaths have long been indicting.

The benefits from naturopathy's other curative standby, 'the waters', have yet to be demonstrated; but after a period while they were unfashionable, they are again attracting custom. Bathing in mineral waters fell into medical disfavour because the standard explanation for their therapeutic usefulness – that beneficient minerals seeped in through the pores of the skin – was shown by experiments in the 1890s to be fallacious. Now, however, it turns out that those experiments were poorly designed. Recent research suggests that not merely is it possible to put therapeutic substances through the skin without breaking it, but that it is actually a safer way than by injection.

Still, whether or not mineral waters are beneficial when applied externally now seems of less significance than it did to the scientists of a century ago. What is important is whether people feel better for them, and how long the improvement lasts. Turkish baths have slipped out of the reckoning, and saunas have tended to pick up a seedy reputation outside their native Finland; but some inland spas continue to appeal to their devotees, and 'thalassotherapy' – sea-water baths, hot and cold, sea-water jets, spurted and sluiced; sea-water and seaweed converted into steam – is being offered at a growing number of establishments around the Continent. The sea, Graupner claimed in his *Adventures in Healing,* 'is the biggest pharmaceutical factory we know,' and for some people it has remarkably rapid therapeutic results. It can be injected; it can be inhaled; it can be drunk (in carefully regulated quantities; shipwrecked sailors die of it only because there is no other source of liquid). And although sea water to drink has yet to catch on, bottled spa water and spring water have recently been enjoying an unprecedented boom, though this may be less for health reasons than because they taste better than recycled sewage from the tap.

Naturopaths are also relishing a further vindication; the sight of medical science retracting its earlier claim that there is no need for bran in the diet. Bran, Michael van Straten, a practitioner of various forms of traditional medicine, has recalled in the *Observer*, used to be 'almost a four-letter word'; when, in 1963, he put a patient on a high-fibre diet her doctor, hearing about it, said he expected it would kill her. But it worked. A decade later research showed that the naturopaths had been right; and the need for 'roughage' has since been firmly established. So, too, has the need for greater care in the marketing of foodstuffs containing colouring matter and preservatives, which naturopaths had been warning against from the start. The extent to which they are responsible for cancer in humans remains to be settled, but their carcinogenic properties have been endlessly demonstrated in laboratory tests with animals.

HERBALISM

Even more than naturopathy, herbalism has appeared to be made obsolete by medical science. If there is any therapeutic substance in a plant, the argument has continued to be, it can be isolated, refined and packaged. Better still, a synthetic product should be produced with the same molecular structure. But this has not always worked in practice, for reasons which are beginning to become apparent.

The way in which doubts arose whether the scientific method really *is* scientific, in this context, is one of the themes of *Herbs that Heal*, by William Thomson. In his preface he is careful to stress that he is not a 'back-to-nature' faddist, but nobody who has followed his career would be likely to harbour that suspicion: he was for many years editor of the medical journal *The Practitioner*, and medical correspondent of *The Times*, as well as being Deputy Chairman of the British Academy of Forensic Sciences. The more he has studied the history of drugs, however, the more he has been forced to recognise that to ignore nature in manufacturing drugs is to ask for trouble. In theory, to extract the 'active principle' of a plant sounds eminently sensible; in the process, impurities can be removed, and therapeutically valueless negative parts of the plant thrown away, or put to some other purpose. But sometimes, in the purification, the 'active principle' appears mysteriously to lose its potency; or it may become too potent. There appears to be 'some braking or balancing mechanism in the plant itself', Thomson suggests, to prevent the active principle from becoming too weak or too powerful.

Among a number of examples Thomson cites the fate of digitalis. It is still, he insists, one of the most valuable drugs in the world pharmacopeia. But too many doctors have stopped using the drug made from the foxglove leaf, having been persuaded by the drug companies' promotion teams to prescribe drugs made from the 'active principle': glycosides. Yet there is no evidence that patients on the glycosides fare better than those on the traditional leaf preparation; and there is ample evidence that treatment with the glycosides is more dangerous, so much so that a Boston doctor has complained that one company's product 'is replacing homicide as a leading cause of death'. In a survey of patients admitted to hospital with heart conditions treated by the glycosides' preparation in most common use, 'One in four was found to be suffering from an overdose of the drug, and of these patients one in sixteen died of digitalis poisoning.'

Encouraged by growing public interest the Society of Herbalists, previously mainly a trading enterprise, decided in 1975 to end its commercial connection, change its name to the Herb Society, and concentrate on research and propaganda to encourage public interest in plants, particularly in connection with disease prevention; and it appointed Malcolm Stuart, a young scientist who had specialised in research into viruses, as director. Stuart had earlier investigated the use of herbs among tribal communities in Africa; and although at first cynical, he was soon convinced that herbalism was a neglected science. His research has led him to believe that in cases like digitalis, 'the whole plant contains secondary effect-enhancing substances, and/or side-effect eliminating substances.' Perhaps they 'buffer' each other, protecting each other from external influences; perhaps they are synergistic, producing effects when they are in combination which they do not have separately; perhaps there are more subtle chemical interactions yet to be unravelled. But whatever the explanation, it can no longer be assumed that isolation of the active ingredient is necessarily the best way to utilise the therapeutic value of a plant; and this has brought the herbalists back into serious contention.

Few tests have been carried out with straightforward herbal remedies. Where they have been held, and it has been shown that the remedies worked, the results have been ignored. In his *Observer* article van Straten recalled that trials in Switzerland in the late 1960s showed that a wide range of plants had the effects which herbalists claimed for them. As antibiotics, diuretics and anti-inflammatory agents they were efficient and safe; and a 'double-blind' trial, with neither the doctors nor the patients knowing which of two groups were receiving the herbal remedy, showed that it brought about a significant reduction in the adverse side-effects of radiation treatment for cancer. But no English hospital could be induced to repeat the experiment.

This prejudice against herbalism may be dying; but most of the money available for such research is distributed either by drug companies, who naturally do not want to promote herbal remedies, or by Foundations, advised by medical scientists conditioned to laboratory investigations of a kind for which plants are not considered suitable. Grown in one garden, plants may have different properties from those grown in a garden in another part of the country. Some herbalists dry herbs and grind them into powder; others make a liquid extract or tincture. Whatever the process, it does not provide the standardised product that medical scientists desire. The impression that treatment with the whole plant can be more effective, as well as safer, than with the 'active principle' consequently has had to rely on evidence of a kind which can easily be dismissed as anecdotal.

Nevertheless it can be striking. A story which attracted wide publicity recently was a case of post-operative infection – increasingly hard to combat, in spite of rigorous measures– in a London hospital, which was treated by strips of the African *Carica Papaya* fruit, 'paw-paw'. The idea came from one of the surgical team, who had seen it used to cure wounds and ulcers in South Africa. Within a week, the infection had cleared up; and although the man died not long after, it was from his original kidney disease, not from the infection. It had not been made clear, the *New Scientist* disparagingly commented, why 'the more orthodox approach of using the fruit's active ingredient (papain) was not adopted'. But the reasons why the less orthodox approach succeeded – apart from coincidence, placebo effect, or auto-suggestion – may turn out to be that the whole fruit is better for healing wounds than its papain.

The problem today, and for the immediate future, is that enormous commercial pressures remain to exploit herbs by isolating the active ingredients, the better to market them; pressures all the greater now that disillusionment is setting in with synthetic laboratory-manufactured drugs. Plants cannot be patented; what the pharmaceutical industry desperately needs is new products derived from plants to maintain its sales, now that 'molecular roulette' is no longer providing them. Some companies have been going to bizarre lengths to find such products, as Thomson describes. *Drosera Rotundifolia*, better known as the sundew, exudes a sticky substance to catch unwary insects, which in Irish folklore has a reputation for soothing sunburn, easing respiratory disorders and promoting fertility in cattle. A German manufacturer, hoping he was on the track of a fortune, and hearing that the sundew is to be found in some bogs, offered to take all the plants the Irish could lay their hands on without giving a thought to the effect this might have on the very delicate ecological balance which the plants help to maintain.

Interviewed for *World Medicine,* Malcolm Stuart has been quoted as saying that his job is 'trying to clear out the mumbo-jumbo and quackery of herbalism'. Can such a line be drawn? One of the 'mumbo-jumbo' beliefs which brought herbalists into contempt was that herbs must be picked not just at some particular season, which was understandable, but at some particular hour. This, Thomson recalls, was held to be hocus-pocus; but 'How wrong those critics have proved to be!' Research has shown that the yield of morphine from poppies early in the morning may be four times the yield in the evening; and a similar variation has been found in the yield of atropine from plants. In other cases, such as the periwinkle – another plant whose existence in its wild state was for a while threatened, when it was found that it had alkaloids that killed white cells in laboratory rats, which led to its being taken up as a possible cure for leukemia – the 'active principle' can be detected only at certain stages of its development. The old herbalists may not always have been correct in their theories or timing, Thomson admits, but 'they knew what they were doing'.

HOMEOPATHY

Neither naturopathy nor herbalism has ever presented a serious threat to medical orthodoxy. Homeopathy did, for a time; but by the 1970s the danger had long since passed. From the ten thousand homeopaths at the beginning of the century, qualifying from twenty medical schools in America, the numbers by the 1970s had shrunk to less than six hundred, and only one medical school remained exclusively homeopathic. There was a similar decline in Britain, in spite of the Royal Family's continued patronage. By the 1970s there were only a hundred medically-qualified homeopaths.

There were two main reasons: the pharmacological revolution – antibiotics, in particular – for a time made homeopathic remedies appear ridiculous; and the fact that the medically-qualified homeopaths had continued to train only medically-qualified entrants so that homeopathy continued to lose many promising recruits, persuaded in the course of their training that it was hopelessly unscientific.

Medical homeopaths sometimes contend that their insistence on the need for full medical training before going on to qualify as a homeopathic practitioner cannot be blamed for what has happened in America and Britain, because there has not been the same decline in France. But in France, homeopathy has remained *the* alternative medicine. Medically-unqualified practitioners have been harassed under the Napoleonic code in ways they cannot be in Britain; and the laws against them have been much more effective than in the United States.

How foolish the homeopaths have been to put their trust in the medical profession – like an antelope seeking sanctuary in the coils of a boa-constrictor – has been illustrated by a recent episode in Liverpool, one of the few cities in Britain where treatment has continued to be available in a homeopathic hospital. Under the 1948 Act setting up the National Health Service, provision was made for the continuance of such homeopathic hospitals as remained. The new regional management committees were to 'maintain the continuity of the characteristics of those institutions', Aneurin Bevan insisted, adding that so far as he was concerned this was an 'absolute guarantee'. But in the course of the re-organisation of the National Health Service in 1974 the regional management committees were axed, leaving the homeopaths with Bevan's pledge but no way to ensure that it was implemented.

When the Department of Homeopathic Medicine in Liverpool was informed that, as part of the general re-organisation, it would be relocated in the new Royal Liverpool Hospital, it resigned itself to making the move. But at a meeting to allocate premises in the new hospital the homeopathic representative was asked to withdraw; and in his absence, the doctors agreed among themselves that the homeopathists must be excluded. They were 'horrified to learn that a Homeopathy clinic was suggested', their Minute ran. They 'insisted unanimously that undergraduates should not be exposed to any unorthodox medicine before qualification; that the very existence of such a clinic in the hospital's prospectus would cause alarm to many doctors and patients; and that the Pharmacy should not be asked to attempt to supply expensive and dangerous remedies'. In the event of their advice being rejected, they agreed, undergraduates would be forbidden to attend the clinic; and they themselves would decline to accept any homeopath as a professional colleague.

Presenting the facts in the House of Commons in 1977 Tom Ellis, MP for Wrexham, suggested that 'for sheer blind prejudice and bigotry, crass ignorance and highly questionable ethical behaviour, it would be hard to find a better example'. But in a sense the homeopaths had asked for it. They had themselves refused to consort with medically-unqualified practitioners. If they were referred to as a branch of alternative medicine (as often they were) they were quick to deny it; in their own eyes, they were *the* alternative. Yet in the eyes of the general public they have always been as much outsiders as the herbalists and the naturopaths. And in the eyes of the medical profession they have been, and still are, not merely outsiders, but outcasts; traitors within the camp.

There would have been more sense in maintaining the link with the medical profession if the homeopaths had been able to exploit it to justify their claims. As the years went by they had come to rely less and less on Hahnemann's theories, and more and more on pragmatism: on the fact that their remedies worked. But when they urged that their remedies should be tested, orthodoxy's reaction was the same as it was to herbalism or manipulation: patients must not be put at risk by being subjected to trials of such a kind. It was not until the mid-1970s that trials were at last laid on, by arrangement between the Centre for Rheumatic Diseases in the Glasgow Royal Infirmary and the Glasgow Homeopathic Hospital, to compare the effect of homeopathic and allopathic remedies in the treatment of rheumatoid arthritis.

Ninety-five patients took part, all of whom fell within the standard diagnostic criteria for 'classical' rheumatoid arthritis and were being treated for it. Forty-one of them, in one group, were given aspirin – still recognised as the most effective and safest form of orthodox treatment, after surviving the promotion campaigns for scores of steroid and anti- inflammatory drugs. The other fifty-four were given homeopathic treatment. Within a few months thirty-five of the aspirin-treated group had dropped out, either because it was doing no good, or because of side-effects. In the same period only fourteen of the homeopathic group dropped out, none of them because of side-effects. By the end of a year six of the aspirin group were clinically better; in the homeopathy group, the number was twenty-four.

From the purists' point of view the trial was inadequately controlled; partly because the patients in the homeopathic group were allowed to continue whatever treatment they had been taking earlier, partly because the two groups were treated by different practitioners, so patients' reaction to them might have influenced the results. Nevertheless the findings are sufficiently clear to undermine the assumption, sedulously propagated for a century and a half, that what the homeopaths think of as 'potentising' their remedies is in fact only diluting them until there is nothing left but water.

There have been other indications that the long decline of homeopathy has been halted. Since 1976 the British Homeopathic Association has reported a massive increase in public enquiries. As has been admitted in the evidence presented to the Royal Commission on the NHS, the demand cannot be met in many parts of the country, because there are no longer homeopathic doctors or clinics and, as a result, patients wanting the treatment have been turning to medically unqualified homeopaths. A few have been in practice for years; but most of them are by training naturopaths, osteopaths, acupuncturists or radiesthetists who have become interested in homeopathy and decided to incorporate it in their range of treatments.

An association has now been formed, the Society of Homeopaths, whose aim is to liberate homeopathy from the dominance of the medical profession, and establish it as 'a complete and independent system of natural therapeutics' with a professional Register of its own and a training college. The reaction of the medically-trained homeopaths to this new development has been frosty; but so long as they cling to the link with the medical profession they cannot hope to meet the new demand, unless they choose to swallow their pride, and come to terms with the newcomers, with a view to acquiring some control over them.

OSTEOPATHY AND CHIROPRACTIC

The chief beneficiaries of the decline of confidence in ortho-dox medicine should have been the osteopaths and chiro-practors, as they were already well-established. In the United States, though, they were if anything *too* well-established. 'In the course of its long struggle for recognition,' Irvin Korr, head of the Physiological Sciences Department at the Kirks-ville College of Osteopathy, has admitted, 'the osteopathic profession appears to have forgotten why it sought recog-nition: to enable it to deliver and demonstrate, as widely as possible, the benefits of osteopathic principles and methods'; and in forgetting, it had permitted osteopathic manipulation 'to slip from its place as a key element in osteopathic practice'.

What has happened is that the medical profession in America has at long last recalled the lesson that homeopathy taught them; that the best way to meet any serious challenge from unorthodoxy is to embrace it and smother it. In 1961 the American Medical Association laid down that it would no longer be an offence to co-operate with osteopaths, because their training was becoming more orthodox; and the follow-ing year two thousand osteopaths in California were awarded medical degrees, their training college being recognised as a medical school. Although osteopaths in other parts of the country have rejected similar proposals for fusion, the trend is clear. Osteopathy will soon cease to be classifiable as alter-native medicine; particularly as reports indicate that osteo-paths are prescribing drugs as freely as, and sometimes more freely, than, physicians.

Chiropractors, too, in America, have been moving in the same direction. By the 1970s chiropractic had been legalised in every State of the Union. But chiropractors do not, as a rule, prescribe drugs, which does a lot to account for the remarkable difference between what they have to pay to in-sure themselves against malpractice suits: on average it is about one-fiftieth of what doctors have now to pay, which incidentally makes nonsense of the stock medical claim that chiropractic is unsafe. To some extent chiropractors have ceased to rely on spinal manipulation, as a comparison between its results and those of orthodox medicine, carried out in Utah, has shown: there was little difference in the chiropractors' methods of treatment, apart from their prescribing fewer drugs, and no significant difference in the results. But in dealing with back trouble their record has been strikingly better than that of the medical profession. A report in 1960 of tests carried out on twenty thousand cases by the Florida Industrial Commission showed that on average, cases handled by doctors cost over twenty-five per cent more; compensation costs were over three hundred per cent more: and loss of working time, under medical treatment, was also around three hundred per cent greater. And comparable studies in the other states have since produced similar findings.

Citing these research findings in the statement to a British Working Group on Back Pain set up by the Ministry of Health, the British Chiropractors' Association has argued that if chiropractic could be made generally available, it must lead to reduced suffering from backache – one of the chief causes of lost working days – and at the same time reduce the overload on existing services and manpower in general practice and in hospitals. But the Association realise it would need to prove the contention in properly controlled clinical trials, involving the co-operation of the medical profession; a course which the Working Group has since recommended in its report.

Sporadic pressure on the medical profession to test manipulation has, in fact, already prompted what was intended as a controlled trial, in the early 1970s with about four hundred and fifty patients divided into four groups, receiving manipulation, physiotherapy, bed-rest or spinal corsets; and when the results showed no significant differences between the manipulated group and the rest they were hailed as a vindication of the profession's refusal to recognise osteopathy. But the trial was poorly designed, as the representatives of the British Association of Manipulative Medicine, all of whose members are doctors, complained at the time; in fact they withdrew from it before it had begun. Their chief objection was that the patients were distributed at random among the groups; anybody who practises manipulation, they argued, selects only patients he thinks will respond. It could also be argued that the test was not of manipulation, and certainly not of osteopathy, but of the skill of an individual manipulator. The trial's most serious defect, though, was that (as is ordinarily the case in such projects) it had been decided not to include results for patients who did not complete the trial. Over a third of those who did not complete it gave as their reason that manipulation had been so successful that they saw no reason to continue with it. Had this figure been included, it would have given manipulation a significant lead over the other standard orthodox treatments, at least in the short term.

ACUPUNCTURE

In orthodox medicine, homeopathy and osteopathy are old antagonists; but acupuncture has presented orthodoxy with a new and baffling problem. How can it be explained away? And how, if it cannot be explained away, can it be fitted into Western-style medicine without the kind of embarrassment that the Vatican would feel if newly discovered Dead Sea scrolls demonstrated the integrity of Judas and Pontius Pilate? Or can it perhaps be accepted but, like hypnotism, relegated to clinical obscurity?

The first instinct of the medical Establishment in Britain – never averse to showing up Americans as over-credulous – was to suggest that although acupuncture might work on a limited scale in China, there had been a lot of fuss about very little. The 1974–5 report of the Medical Research Council, notoriously wedded to investigation along strictly orthodox lines, claimed that only a small percentage of patients in China responded to acupuncture analgesia; and even for them, days of preparation were required, lengthening the time of hospitalisation and increasing the cost of surgery. Acupuncture would consequently be suitable for only a small proportion of surgical cases in Britain because it involved uncertainties which would be unacceptable.

There was a measure of truth in the commentary, particularly in the reference to uncertainty. But it was chiefly concerned with the consequences of any attempt to introduce acupuncture in British hospitals as an alternative to anesthetics; and this was unlikely to happen, except on a small scale for experimental purposes. For use in the treatment of, say, arthritis or headache, no protracted preparation is required, and treatment is less expensive than that with conventional drugs.

But is it more effective? The other view expressed by many Western observers was that if acupuncture works, it must work by placebo-effect, reinforced by auto-suggestion and perhaps by some form of hypnosis. But the results of trials conducted with controls, some patients receiving traditional acupuncture and others having needles stuck into them at places not indicated in the old Chinese charts, led the *British Medical Journal* to admit early in 1977 that acupuncture had been shown to be 'significantly more effective than suggestion' in raising the threshold at which patients began to feel pain.

Such results, though, have sometimes been equivocal. It is as if auto-suggestion, or perhaps the rapport between the acupuncturist and patient, supplements the effect of the needles, and doubtless in some circumstances does their work for them, as a dummy pill can do the work of an opiate. That some patients react differently to acupuncture according to mood has long been recognised in China, and it is confirmed by research in Europe, where it has been found that people respond less well who are suffering from anxiety. But it is no longer seriously disputed that some process other than suggestion is involved. Various theories have been put forward: that the spinal cord has a 'gate' mechanism activated by the needles to restrict the flow of impulses through the nervous system: that acupuncture is a version of a method of pain relief long known in folk-lore, where a short sharp pain is supposed to bring relief from protracted chronic pain; or that acupuncture is a way of activating and encouraging the manufacture and distribution of certain pain-reducing substances, comparable to opiates, which the body itself manufactures. No theory, though, has yet been found wholly acceptable; and the possibility still remains that some as yet unexplained force is involved.

One thing has become clear: the results of 'controlled' trials are so varied that they cast doubts on the reliability of standard control procedures. Occasionally they are almost too good to be acceptable. In New Orleans fifty volunteers were randomly assigned to receive either acupuncture or a local anesthetic before dentists drilled their teeth (though as a precaution, it was agreed that a patient could at any time indicate his dissatisfaction with acupuncture, and revert to a local anesthetic). According to the report presented to the American Society of Anesthesiologists, ninety per cent of those who tried acupuncture said they felt no more pain than they would have expected to feel if they had been given an anesthetic. Even more significant, with one exception they said that if they were given the choice they would prefer acupuncture on their next visit to the dentist.

Other trials have provided much less encouraging results. Yet what has transpired is that for some types of disorder common in the West acupuncture offers hope where all orthodox remedies have failed. This has perhaps best been expressed in the report of tests conducted in a hospital in Buffalo, New York, and published in 1976 in *Advances in Pain Research and Therapy*. Eighty-seven patients suffering from chronic pain were given an average of eight treatments; half of them obtained no lasting benefit, and only one third still felt better three months later. A negative view of these results, the report observed, would be that, at least for American patients, acupuncture is a costly, time-consuming and painful procedure, helping only a minority. But 'A positive view of the same results would emphasise that of a sample of patients with chronic pain who had not obtained significant relief with a variety of traditional forms of treatment, about one-third obtained moderate to complete relief.' And as Ronald Melzack of McGill University, one of the inventors of the 'gate' theory, remarked after a trial there which had a comparable effect, 'Even a few hours or days of pain at tolerable levels permits some patients to live with more dignity and self-assurance.'

The chief problem, though, for anybody seeking acupuncture has been to find it. In the United States, as soon as the AMA had recovered from the shock of hearing that acupunc-

ture worked, it was quick to heed Dimond's advice and insist
that nobody other than a doctor (or an osteopath) would be
allowed to give it; by 1975 only one State, Nevada, permitted
acupuncturists who were not doctors to treat patients. As
there were only a handful of doctors in the entire country
who were acupuncturists, this meant handing acupuncture over
to people who had no experience of, and previously no interest
in, the treatment; and although doctors were permitted to employ an acupuncturist without medical qualification, provided
he was kept under 'direct supervision', few of them had sufficient experience of acupuncture or its practitioners for such
supervision to be adequate. Acupuncturists, qualified or self-
taught, soon began to break the law, and many prosecutions
have followed.

In Britain the medically-unqualified practitioners have been
better placed to take advantage of the renewed demand; and
in this they have been assisted by the continued refusal of the
medical acupuncturists to allow anybody other than a doctor
to undertake their course of training. As a result, the number
of medically-qualified acupuncturists has remained very small.

RADIESTHESIA

In November 1973 British television viewers who had been
watching the election of that year's 'Miss World' and who
had not switched off their sets, were treated to what was either
the most remarkable display of conjuring, or the first display
of the power of the mind over matter, that they had ever
seen: cutlery bent, and the minute hands of watches twisted
into strange shapes. Uri Geller divided the community into
believers and sceptics, as his performances all over the world
have done ever since; but what cannot be disputed is that he
introduced the subject of paranormal phenomena into the
living rooms of millions. And not only the living rooms; by
the hundred, viewers and newspaper readers wrote in to say
that kitchen cutlery had bent, and hall-way clocks which had
long been out of action had started to tick, or chime, while he
was performing.

What Geller could do, assuming that he was genuinely

possessed of psychic powers, did not appear to have any immediate relevance to healing. But on reflection, people who had been involved or become interested in any form of healing which could not be accounted for in orthodox terms began to realise its significance. If matter could be distorted in this way by psychic emanations – not necessarily from Geller himself : he might have triggered them off in viewers – the whole of medical history would need to be reassessed, and large portions of it rewritten. Shamanism and witchcraft, if not accounted for, would at least be brought closer to some rational explanation; perhaps even in terms scientists could accept.

Of the vitalist theories which were still practised, the one which appeared to have most to gain from the discovery of such an explanation – or at least acceptance of the reality of the phenomena, even if they could not be explained – was radiesthesia, along with its radionic devices. On the theoretical side, radiesthesists had already been given cause for satisfaction by the discoveries of the nuclear physicists, who had been demolishing the materialist structure on which nineteenth century science had been based. It was no longer possible to dismiss psychokinetic action at a distance as against the laws of nature; on the contrary, the ability of atomic particles to move from one orbit to another without traversing the intervening space – dematerialising, as it were, and re-materialising – and to mimic other paranormal manifestations has led the French physicist Costa de Beauregard to assert that so far as quantum mechanics is concerned, 'Phenomena such as psychokinesis or telepathy, far from being irrational, should on the contrary be expected as very rational.' What radiesthesists had previously lacked, though, was a demonstration of the ability of the mind to act on matter, showing people – those, at least, who were willing to accept Geller as genuine – how radiesthesia might work.

In particular, acceptance of 'the Geller effect' bridged the incredulity gap which had worried many people who might otherwise have been sympathetic to radiesthesia. The idea that a blood sample might carry in it information about the health of a distant patient was not too difficult to accept; a believer in extra-sensory perception could regard the sample simply as a tuning mechanism, whereby the mind of the radiesthesist was connected by telepathy or clairvoyance with the patient. But it had been harder to credit the idea of health-giving transmissions winging their way back to the patient by courtesy of the radionic 'box'. Yet Horder and his colleague, fifty years before, had both felt something happening in their diaphragms when the experiments were in progress, as if they were receiving the message internally. If psychokinetic transmissions were not significantly affected by distance, there would be no reason to reject the possibility that they, too, could make themselves felt, however far away the patient might be.

Acceptance that a psychic element is involved has also meant that radiesthesists no longer need to provide evidence that their radionic gadgets can make an objective diagnosis of the kind Abrams, Drown and de la Warr tried so hard to demonstrate. This has been much to the relief of practitioners such as Frances Farrelly, the best known of the American radiesthesists. Becoming interested in the subject while working as a medical technician Farrelly took a course with Ruth Drown; and while working with her noticed that occasionally when they were testing a sample of blood somebody had sent in, they would get results, only to find when they came to remove the sample that they had forgotten to put it in the machine. Clearly, Farrelly realised, the instruments themselves were *not* doing the work. And this has now come to be more generally accepted. Most radionic practitioners regard the 'box', or whatever it is they use, as the equivalent of the dowser's pendulum or hazel twig. A few of them believe that the device can absorb psychic energy, so that it will be capable of facilitating diagnosis and treatment in much the same way as an object can give information to a medium by 'psychometry'; but the medium remains indispensable.

Farrelly restricts herself to diagnosis, from her Florida home; if she diagnosed and treated patients she would be breaking the law. Blood samples are sent to her from all over the country; and for each one she goes into what she takes to be an altered state of consciousness – not a trance, as she remains aware of what is going on around her – but an abstracted condition. By focussing her attention on the blood sample, she finds, she can obtain a diagnosis. In other words she does what tribal doctors have traditionally done, and what scores of psychics and mediums have been reported as doing throughout history; using extra-sensory perception for divination, with or without aids.

But does her method work? The presumption must be that it does, as she is employed by over seventy doctors, some of whom have sent her blood samples for ten years or more. They would not have continued to send them, presumably, if her diagnoses did not score above chance level. Still, it would obviously be more satisfactory if her results, and those of other radiesthesists, could be checked in formal tests.

The problem here has been that doctors who employ a radiesthesist are rarely willing to admit as much; and even the prospect of exposing radiesthesia as a superstition or a fraud has not always been a sufficient inducement to persuade sceptics to co-operate in formal trials. In the United States there have also been legal problems. In Britain the sceptics have it both ways: on the one hand they have said that radiesthesia cannot work, and is consequently not worth testing; on the other, when Alec Forbes suggested a trial in Plymouth it was turned down on the excuse that it would be unethical to subject patients to such treatment.

In any case, most practitioners are wary of the kind of tests they would be likely to be asked to do. They do not expect to be consistently right in their diagnostic role (any more than doctors do); and they feel that they are more likely to be wrong in test conditions in which, they claim, they find it hard to reach the altered state of consciousness – the abstracted condition – in which they perform most confidently. They can reasonably point out, too, that failures of the kind that damaged Ruth Drown's reputation are remembered, while Boyd's spectacular success when tested by the Horder committee is forgotten. The only satisfactory method of testing, they argue, would be to monitor their results over a period of months, or even years; and this has yet to be tried.

One form of testing, though, is occasionally reported:

usually the work of some joker. The medical editor of *General Practitioner*, David Delvin, sent a couple of hairs to a member of the British Radionics Association in 1977, along with a case history which indicated that he was a diabetic; and when the radiesthesist failed to recognise that they came from a cat, Delvin was able to mock him in an article in *World Medicine*. As it happened, though, Delvin had to admit that the radiesthesist's diagnosis, 'very overstrained' was not far off the mark; the cat had just been neutered.

The test was in any case misguided. In trials over a six-year period Gertrude Schmeidler, Professor of Psychology at the City College, New York, had earlier established that people who believe in (or at least accept the possibility of) extra-sensory perception score higher than chance expectation, on balance, in tests designed to discover if they have ESP; whereas sceptics score lower. Paradoxically, these results can be held to demonstrate the existence of ESP; if it does not exist, both sets of scores ought to have been at the same chance level. From this and much supporting evidence it has come to be accepted by parapsychologists that sceptics can exert a 'negative' influence. If so, tests carried out by sceptics like Delvin which appear to invalidate radiesthesia may simply be validating their own psychic power – hardly what they are anxious to prove.

HEALING

In 1961 an article appeared in the *International Journal of Parapsychology* which had some claim to be a report of the first scientific investigation into healing. Up to that time the medical Establishments had effectively blocked such research: either, as in Britain, through the threat of erasure hanging over any doctor who sent patients to a medically-unqualified practitioner; or, as in the United States, by the rule that doctors must not associate professionally with anyone whose treatment was not 'founded on a scientific basis'. Biochemists, however, were not subject to the same sanctions; and Bernard Grad of McGill University had an idea for an experiment which, as it happened, got round both obstacles: it was scientific, and it did not involve patients.

Grad's aim was to discover whether healing by 'the laying-on of hands' was effective, and if so, whether it could be attributed to suggestion. As his healer he had Colonel Estebany, a former Hungarian army officer who had discovered he had healing powers and had continued to use them (though not professionally; because he believed he was merely the channel through which the healing flowed from a divine source, he would take no fee). And as his patients Grad had laboratory mice.

In the first test, the mice were anesthetised so that small 'nicks' could be made in their backs, and were then divided into three evenly-matched groups. Ordinarily, a single control group would have sufficed; but as Grad realised that if the experiment succeeded it could be suggested that the healing might have been due to a change of temperature, the cage of one of the two control groups of mice was heated to a degree sufficient to match the warmth from Estebany's hands. Estebany held the underside of his cage of mice with one hand, putting his other hand over the top of it; and the backs of the mice which he treated healed significantly faster than the backs of the mice in either of the control groups. To make sure that some unexplained experimenter-effect was not involved, a further trial was then carried out 'double blind', nobody knowing which group of mice was which until after it had ended, and with the additional precaution that another group of mice were given Estebany-type treatment, but not by a healer. The results were the same as in the first test: Estebany's set of mice healed faster than the other sets.

Further experiments followed, using seeds; Estebany showing that he could influence their growth rate not only by holding his hands over the seeds, but also by holding the bottle out of which they were watered. Even more remarkable results were obtained by the research scientist Robert N. Miller of Atlanta, in controlled tests of a similar nature, but of 'distant healing'; from their home in Baltimore Ambrose and Olga Worrall, by concentrating on their objective, managed to increase the growth rate of rye grass in Miller's laboratory, six hundred miles away, by over eight hundred per cent, the growth being recorded on a strip chart. And in 1967 it occurred to Justa Smith that the same kind of experiments could be undertaken with enzymes, bringing the research a stage closer to man.

A Franciscan nun, Justa Smith was also an experienced bio-chemist, with a doctorate for her research into the effects of magnetism on enzymes; and she decided to compare the effect of the laying-on of hands – Estebany, again, was brought in – with the known effect of magnetism. The controls were similar to those of the Grad experiments, and the results were even more impressive. Estebany's hands had the same effect on enzyme activity as a magnetic field 150,000 times more powerful than normal; yet there was no trace of a magnetic field between his hands.

As enzymes are capable of acting as catalysts, facilitating chemical changes within the body, Justa Smith's findings were of great significance for the medical profession. Yet the *New England Journal of Medicine,* the *British Medical Journal* and other prestigious publications ignored them; thereby drawing down a rebuke from Geoff Watts, Deputy Editor of *World Medicine.* It might, he feared, be no more than a manifestation 'of the same set of prejudices which has already determined our own attitudes to the "scientific" and "unscientific" '; the fact that such reports are rejected on grounds of unorthodoxy, therefore, 'should not be allowed to add weight to our dis-belief'. But *World Medicine* in this period (the early 1970s) was one of the few medical journals of standing in which Justa Smith's work would have even been mentioned, unless she had succeeded in showing that Estebany had concealed a high-powered magnet under his finger-nails, in which case she could have expected an editorial pat on her head.

It was becoming increasingly difficult, though, for medical journals to ignore the results of research into healing; and in June 1973 John Carlova, senior editor of *Medical Economics,* reported that Olga Worrall's powers had been tested at a con-ference of doctors and scientists at Stanford University. She had been invited to heal ten patients for whom the resources of orthodox treatment had been exhausted; and seven out of

the ten, according to their doctors, were either cured or benefitted from her laying-on of hands. The experiment was on too
small and informal a scale to be acceptable as evidence of her
healing: what was significant was that it had been conducted
at a gathering of that kind.

Some tests of healers' diagnostic powers have been undertaken, too, with interesting results. The neurologist Norman
Shealy invited three clairvoyant healers to his Wisconsin clinic;
and after seeing the patients, without being allowed to talk to
them or know anything about them, the clairvoyants correctly
diagnosed what was the matter with them four times out of five
(one of the healers, like the psychic investigated by the French
Academies' commission a century and a half before, actually
contradicted Shealy's own diagnosis: correctly, it later transpired). Realising that the controls would need to be more
rigorous if the results were to be acceptable, Shealy then did a
further series of tests in which the psychics were not allowed
to see the patients; they worked from photographs. They were
asked to locate in which of twenty-two areas of their bodies
seventy patients were suffering pain. As a precaution, a professor of psychology with no pretensions to psychic abilities acted
as a one-man control group; and he duly scored at around
chance level, with five to ten per cent correct results. The
three clairvoyants correctly named the source of the pain in
seventy to seventy-five per cent of the cases, and the location
of the pain in between sixty and sixty-five percent. As Shealy
observed, this rate is not far off what a competent doctor
would expect to achieve using modern equipment; and high
enough to suggest that psychics could give valuable assistance
in cases where there is diagnostic uncertainty.

The scientific evidence that an unexplained healing power
exists, coupled with the mass of historical examples, has become strong enough to convince many doubters in the medical
profession, so that they no longer feel humiliated when
patients admit that they have sought a healer's help. But it
has taken so long for healing to achieve this limited recognition that it has been largely appropriated by religious sects.
During the past fifty years the Spiritualists and various pentecostal groups have increasingly come to regard healing as an

essential feature of their services; and according to a report in the *New York Times* in the summer of 1978 spiritual healing has been 'rapidly gaining favour' even in staid Episcopalian churches, more than fifteen hundred of which now hold a weekly healing service.

Healing is also, the report claimed, attracting more interest in Catholic circles. The Vatican has remained suspicious, as its treatment of the Capucin 'Padre Pio' showed: when in 1918 he began to suffer from the stigmata, and the news sent pilgrims flocking to his monastery near Foggia, every effort was made to prevent him from becoming a cult figure over the remaining fifty years of his life, in spite of many well-attested reports of miracles attributed to him. And although Lourdes has been allowed to continue as a healing centre, attracting millions of pilgrims every year, the number of miraculous cures accepted by the Church has continued to dwindle; from 1962 to 1975 the committee of doctors set up to adjudicate in possible cases was convened on only five occasions. According to the *Times* report, however, healing services in Catholic Churches in America have risen spontaneously, often without reference to the authorities; and they are becoming ecumenical, with Catholics and Episcopalians joining in the 'Charismatic movement', as it has come to be known.

All over the world, too, there are individuals who exercise healing powers of a kind which cannot be adequately explained by suggestion and auto-suggestion, though they may play their part. Often they remain unknown, except to friends. Some attract a devoted following, as Madame Sikora, a Polish refugee 'magnetiser' and clairvoyant, did in London in the 1960s. In *The Realms of Healing* Stanley Krippner, an experienced investigator of paranormal phenomena, and Alberto Villoldo describe the work of others who have achieved national fame: 'Rolling Thunder' in the United States, Fausto Valle in Peru, Joseph Zezulka in Prague. And as the British psychoanalyst Joan Fitzherbert noted in a paper on the nature of hypnosis and paranormal healing in 1971, there are some cases where apparently instantaneous cures are attested by the doctors of the patients concerned, including two credited to the Pittsburgh healer Kathryn Kuhlman: one of a massive goitre which simply vanished in the course of a healing service; another which 'required the instantaneous development of a sizeable piece of new bone'. In such cases, proof positive is not possible, because the patient has not been subjected to what scientists would regard as adequate controls. Retrospectively, too, it is always possible to bring up 'rational' explanations. But after a time, the rational explanations can become harder to accept than the possibility that some healing force has been in operation.

Chapter Eight

THE PROBLEMS

In retrospect, natural medicine can reasonably be claimed to have been less destructive than mechanistic medicine. Such scientific research as there has been suggests that the community would run no serious risks if naturopathy, herbalism, osteopathy, chiropractic, acupuncture, radiesthesia and healing were recognised as valid forms of treatment and made available, for anybody who wishes to use them, within the health services of their nations. And although health services are not as a rule geared to absorb them, there are many indications that their assistance would now be gratefully received.

To doctors they would be welcome chiefly because they would syphon off patients for whom orthodox medicine can do little except prescribe psychotropic drugs – sedatives, tranquillisers and anti-depressants. Year after year the medical journals sound the alarm about the over-prescribing of these drugs; year after year the number of psychotropic drugs prescribed has continued to increase, not because doctors want to prescribe them, but because patients become increasingly dependent upon them. Some opposition can be expected to any scheme designed to bring medically-unqualified practitioners into a health service without subjecting them to the profession's control; but the reaction would not now be violent, unless they were allowed to treat patients in hospitals.

Even medical scientists, who would ordinarily be expected to man the barricades against intruders, are less actively hostile than they were a decade ago. 'The undoubted successes of acupuncturists, herbalists, osteopaths and other exponents of alternative medicine frequently bear witness to the failure of conventional therapy,' Bernard Dixon, editor of the *New Scientist,* has admitted in *Beyond the Magic Bullet*; and this, he feels, is leading to 'a growing tolerance (at least) by scientific medicine of these heterodox disciplines'.

In the past, governments have tended to allow the medical profession to dictate their attitude to alternative medicine; but they are now aware that they no longer have so much to fear from confrontation on this issue. The British Department of Health, in particular, has begun to realise the advantages of widening the scope of the National Health Service. In 1978 Marcus McCausland, founder of the 'Health for the New Age' organisation, persuaded the Minister, David Ennals, to attend a small conference so that he could hear the views of some representatives of such bodies as the British Committee for Natural Therapeutics, the Healing Research Trust, the Scientific and Medical Network and the Association for Humanistic Psychology; and when later in the year Ennals received the report of the working party on back pain, he expressed his satisfaction that it had recommended tests of osteopathy, chiropractic and acupuncture, and also that the General Medical Council had stated that it would have no ethical objections if, subject to the usual safeguards for patients, the agency set up to control the trials included unorthodox practitioners as well as doctors. 'We cannot afford to disregard or condemn any form of treatment which is demonstrably efficacious,' Ennals commented, 'even if there is, as yet, some uncertainty about why it is efficacious'; an attitude neatly condensed by a headline writer on the *Scotsman* into 'Minister backs quacks'.

Perhaps even more encouraging, in the long term, has been the change of attitude in the World Health Organisation over the past decade. It was a stubbornly conventional body until, in the late 1960s, the recruits from the developing countries began to manifest dissatisfaction with Western-style medicine, and particularly with its bland assumption that it had nothing to learn from tribal ways. After preliminary sparring a joint UNICEF/WHO report in 1974 recommended that the services of practitioners of traditional medicine should, where possible, be utilised in primary health care, a recommendation accepted by the executive of WHO in 1975. The following year a working group was set up in Geneva to assist in the development of traditional medicine, and to seek to combine its knowledge and skills with those of the West.

At first the emphasis was mainly on the need to use traditional medicine either where trained doctors, hospitals and drugs were not available, or where they were available only at an unacceptably high cost. But it soon became apparent that tribal medicine had something to teach orthodoxy. Introducing an article headlined 'New Respectability for "Witch Doctors"' in the summer of 1978, the *New Scientist* referred to 'dramatic shifts in international thinking', which meant that 'the former untouchable of the medical profession, the traditional healer' was achieving recognition.

The significance of this change of attitude has been grasped by paramedical practitioners in Europe. WHO, they realise, could be a useful ally in their dealing with their governments, and still more in their dealings with the European Economic Community. The International Federation of Practitioners of Natural Therapeutics, set up in Britain in 1965 to try to deal with the problems likely to arise out of Britain's entry into the EEC, has approached WHO with a view to establishing a relationship; and although the Federation has suffered from internal wrangles, and WHO's regulations stipulate a probationary period before any formal connection can be made, there seems every likelihood that paramedical practitioners will eventually achieve recognition.

DISUNITY

On the face of it, therefore, the prospects for traditional medicine have been transformed; the Cinderella of the 1950s awaits only the arrival of the Fairy Godmother to take her place in the gravy train. But there is no Fairy Godmother; Cinders still lives in Hard-up Hall; the broker's men are still lurking round the corner. None of the organisations is in funds; none has much prospect of attracting them for development, organisation or research. Enormous sums are pumped into medical organisations each year by the pharmaceutical industry, for purposes ranging from serious investigations to 'conferences' or 'seminars' which are often no more than lavish holidays in the sun or on the golf course. The practitioners of traditional medicine do not, and cannot hope to, enjoy such perks.

It is also difficult for practitioners who are just beginning to obtain recognition, financial as well as clinical, to spare the time to attend to organisational matters, largely at their own expense. They are not even sustained by the expectation that their time will be considered well spent by the practitioners of other therapies, or even of their own. The setting-up of an institutional framework within which traditional medicine can operate is complicated by the existence of internal divisions, and sometimes of feuds.

An indication of the difficulties was given in 1973, when a meeting was held at the House of Commons under the Joint Chairmanship of two MP's, the former Transport Minister Ernest Marples and Joyce Butler. It had been arranged in order to give representatives of various organisations, collected under the umbrella of 'Natural Therapeutics' a chance to express their fears that if Britain should enter the European Economic Community, as was planned, the way would be open for the introduction of restrictive regulations alien to British custom, but established in France under the Napoleonic code.

Marples agreed that the prospect of Britain entering the EEC was a reasonable cause for concern; and he suggested that the best way to ensure that unorthodox practices were protected would be for Natural Therapeutics to secure statutory recognition. But this, he warned, could only be obtained if its practitioners could form a united front; a single organisation representing all branches. And how slim the prospects of all the branches getting together to form a trunk, let alone put down the necessary roots, was clear from the composition of the meeting. The medically-unqualified homeopaths had not been invited, because they lacked an organisation (the medical homeopaths would not have come if they had been asked, believing they would not need protection). The healers had not been invited because at that time they were not considered an integral part of the Natural Therapeutic scene. And the organisations which were represented were not, or not necessarily, representative of all the practitioners within each putative discipline. Most of them had dissident elements; some were fragmented. No fewer than four different osteopathic organisations had been invited to send representatives; the largest of them had declined, ostensibly because it did not feel that the time was ripe for such an approach but also, the other osteopaths suspected, because of resentment at the fact that they had been invited too.

DIVISIONS

There have always been, and doubtless will continue to be, such divisions within the movement. They arise from a number of causes, one being that practitioners of unorthodox methods who are members of the medical profession have tended not merely to keep their distance from medically-unqualified practitioners, but also to be scathing about them.

In 1939 Dr Guyon Richards and a small group of doctors formed the Medical Society for the Study of Radiesthesia; a courageous venture at that time, as it could do a doctor's reputation nothing but harm if his colleagues or his patients knew he was mixed up in anything so dubious. Some of its members, notably Tertius Watson, Aubrey Westlake, and Michael Ash, made important contributions to the literature on the subject. But they found they could exercise no perceptible influence within their profession, and much less than they might have exercised among medically-unqualified radiesthetists (except by their writings); and gradually the society ceased to function. Yet when a new group was formed in 1968 by a surgeon and a dentist, its membership, too, was confined to members of the medical and dental professions on the ground that radiesthesia in the past had been 'strewn with increasing numbers of unfortunate people who have strayed into a cloud-cuckoo-land of fantasy', demonstrating 'the inherent dangers of the use of the pendulum without recourse to valid knowledge'. The implicit assumption that members of the medical profession have a monopoly of valid knowledge was all the more eccentric in view of the fact that nine out of ten doctors, if asked, would have had no hesitation in saying that radiesthesia was not merely invalid, but either crazy or fraudulent.

The common excuse for such groups is that only by keeping themselves free from contamination by outsiders can they hope to influence their professional colleagues. It has never worked: nor have expedients such as, in this case, calling themselves 'The Psionic Medical Society' to avoid the implications of 'radionics'. Name changing of this kind is counter-productive; the proliferation of different terms simply makes for more misunderstanding and more mistrust.

The medical acupuncturists, homeopaths and manipulators, too, by their dog-in-the-consulting-room attitude, have in the recent past deprived themselves of the opportunity to assist, and at the same time to exercise some control over, what is taught and practised by their counterparts. Their enforced apartheid has also been indirectly responsible for divisions within the ranks of the outsiders. British osteopaths who have done their training in the United States, for example, maintain their own separate association in the forlorn hope that in Britain, as in the US, they will be recognised by the medical profession. When they set up a training college, they enrolled only doctors as students (too few applied for the venture to flourish); and they have declined to have any formal links with the main British osteopathic body, practitioners who qualify through the British School of Osteopathy.

Qualification through the School brings a diploma (with the right to put 'DO' after the name) and a place in the Osteopathic Register (with the right to put 'MRO' after the name), a system introduced on the advice of the Ministry of Health as a way of gaining public confidence by enabling people to recognise trained osteopaths. But it has also meant that osteopaths who have qualified by another training course to become members of the British Naturopathic and Osteopathic Association do not get on to the Register because the School of

Osteopathy, which in effect controls the Register, has refused to recognise their qualifications; so they put 'MBNOA' after their names – except for a breakaway group whose members, feeling that too little emphasis was being placed upon osteopathy in the training, have formed their own Society of Osteopaths, calling themselves 'MSO'. There is also the College of Osteopathy, which claims to have the highest training standards of all and includes chiropractors among its members, who style themselves 'FCO'.

DO; MRO; MBNOA; MSO; FCO – until very recently most GP's regarded the lot of them as bogus. Many still do. Certainly the proliferation of capital letters does nothing to fulfil its object: to provide both the profession and the public with reassurance that the practitioner has satisfied his examiners, and remains subject to his association's disciplinary code.

Formal qualifications can in any case be of doubtful relevance in the practice of natural medicine, as Herbert Barker's career showed. The ability of a healer cannot be satisfactorily measured by any known form of examination. And even if the method by which students qualify were to be left flexible, each discipline having its own system, this would lead to further disputes, such as those which break out between purists and pragmatists. Purists insist on maintaining the ideas of the founder – Hahnemann, or Still, or Palmer, or whoever he may be – unsullied; pragmatists feel it is foolish to assume that what the founder wrote is the last word that can ever be said on the subject. The rules of the Incorporated Society of Registered Naturopaths, established in 1927, actually laid down that members must not use other forms of treatment, with the result that the Society has only had a score or so of active practitioners. Most naturopaths have been members of the more flexible BNOA, many of them practising not only naturopathy and osteopathy, but herbalism, homeopathy and acupuncture, suiting treatment to their own and their patients' preferences.

Perhaps the commonest of all causes of disruption, though, are personality clashes. Any individual who has made a success of his career in what until quite recently was a depressed area of therapeutics is likely to have done so by force of personality and through faith in his own theories and practices. He is consequently apt to feel that anybody who favours some rival theory or practice must be wrong, and perhaps dishonest. Often, too, there is a showman element in such individuals, just as there has often been in the men who rise to plush consulting rooms in Harley Street. And though it attracts patients, in colleagues it frequently breeds mistrust.

DIVERSITY

Divisions of all these kinds, actual or potential, make it hard for the practitioners of alternative medicine to reach agreement among themselves, let alone to give a mandate to anybody or any group to negotiate on their behalf. But even if they could be persuaded to sink their differences, there is a further problem which becomes more difficult to deal with every year. Natural medicine has always thrown out offshoots. Some keep in the public eye; some are preserved only by tiny groups of devotees; some disappear. Dissatisfaction with orthodox medicine, as well as improving the prospects for the established therapies, has led to the revival of others which had seemed moribund. Some of them will fade away again; but if natural medicine is going to be brought into health services, it will need to be able to accommodate any of them which expand, as a few show signs of doing.

At first sight they appear to be too heterogeneous to classify; but most of them fall into five main categories (though there is considerable overlapping): nature cure; acupuncture derivatives; refinements or extensions of manipulation and massage; psychic healing; and new versions of psychotherapy, some with an element of mysticism. Their therapeutic merit is hard to evaluate; in each of them it depends more on the ability of the practitioner than on the treatment – and even more, probably, on the degree of rapport which is established with the patient. But they are all now available in Western countries.

NATURE CURE

The most commonly encountered forms of treatment related
to nature cure are those concerned with diet, from vegetarian-
ism to macrobiotics; familiar enough everywhere. But there
are some movements which have only recently surfaced, designed to produce a harmony of mind and body through
neglected or under-developed sensory faculties, such as rhythm
and music can provide.

The historical significance of music therapy was emphasised
almost a hundred and fifty years ago by J. G. Millingen in his
Curiosities of Medical Experience. Saul's madness, he recalled,
had been relieved by David's performance on the harp, and
Pythagoras had prescribed music for mental disorders in
general; it had also been quite extensively used in classical
times to cure fevers, and even as a way of warding off plagues.
Later it continued to be used mainly for the treatment of
mania, though occasionally a doctor would suggest it might
have a wider application; Samuel Johnson's physician, Richard
Brocklesby, thought it could 're-establish the former union of
the body and mind', so that even if it were not, strictly-speak-
ing, medicinal, it would enable proper medicines to 'be administered to better purpose'. In his *Adventures in Healing*
Graupner described how music had been used in a German
health resort to treat psychosomatic disorders such as
stomach ulcers; and Roberto Assagioli has devoted a chapter
to the subject in his *Psychosynthesis*, giving detailed advice in
how music can be used for psycho-physiological rather than
aesthetic purposes. The chief problem, he admits, is that not
only do people react differently to the same piece of music (in
an experiment with over one thousand subjects, half were
shown to find Wagner's 'Ride of the Valkyries' joyous and
stimulating; a third found it irritating and agitating), but the
same individual may react differently according to mood;
'cheerful music may jar on a person weighed down by grief'.

The medical profession makes little use of music therapy,
except in a few mental hospitals; it has chiefly been taken up
by practitioners of alternative medicine, sometimes in conjunction with dance therapy. Here, too, there is a long histori-

cal tradition. Dancing was one of the standard therapeutic techniques of shamanism, designed to provide the tribe, or individuals, with a kind of psycho-physiological saturnalia; and it seems likely that a frenzied dance like the tarantella, though it was attributed to mania brought on by the bite of the tarantula spider, originally had the same purpose. Today the aim is 'to make the individual cognizant of his feelings through the direct sensation of movement', as a practitioner describes it in Mark Bricklin's *Encyclopedia of Natural Healing*. 'By translating emotional conflict into movement, problems become concrete'; the goal being a re-integration of mind and body. There is an American Dance Therapy Association which lays down guidelines, though it admits that they are extremely flexible.

Recently the dance therapy tradition has been reinforced from the East. Legend had it that 'T'ai Chi' originated in Taoist monasteries as a way of keeping children from becoming restless; but it came to be used as a way to achieve the most effective and economical co-ordination of mind and body through exercises designed to ensure that they work in harmony. It is more easily demonstrated than described, resembling as it does a protracted ballet (though its practitioners prefer to think of it as 'moving meditation') combining formalised self-defence with the exercising of all parts of the body, all done in slow, or at least leisurely motion; the aim being to release untapped reserves of 'Chi' – psychic energy. In the process the restraints which mind and body exercise over each other are broken down so that, as one of the leading practitioners, Mrs Gerda Geddes has put it, 'One appears to be living in an open body which seems to be filled with light and air.'

'Aikido' is a less balletic version of T'ai Chi: 'The teacher speaks about harmony, and then throws the student to the ground.' But the aim is the same, or so its teachers assert. By alternatively throwing and being thrown in a series of controlled movements, the student learns that life is not for the strong but for those whose physical strength is combined with 'Chi' – the psychic energy dimension, which gives him better control over his life and health.

Two other forms of therapy fall into this category. In early civilisations oils were extensively used in medical treatment: to promote healing (the good Samaritan poured oil on the wounds of the man who fell among thieves); to facilitate massage; and to provide psychic or spiritual protection ('the Lord's anointed'). It was also believed that the aroma from oils provided strength; athletes performed the better for it, and lovers were recommended to use them not just for the sensual pleasure, but because the perfumes were aphrodisiacs. Later, sniffing them was believed to give protection from the plague. Recently 'aromatherapy' has been reviving. The oils are not of the kind associated with the kitchen or the garage; they are distilled from the substances which give plants and flowers their odour. They are rubbed into the skin, usually in conjunction with massage or manipulation, partly for the purpose long advertised and provided by beauty parlours to refresh or 'tone-up' the skin, partly in the belief that breathing in the aroma tones up the system as a whole.

There is also colour therapy, first advocated in its present form by Edwin Bobbet in the United States a century ago. It is derived from the realisation that most people react to colours emotionally, as well as esthetically; finding some shades soothing, others disturbing. Treatment consists of eliciting individual reactions to colours and using them either to stimulate or soothe, according to need; and also to help people to become more aware of their reactions so that they learn to avoid, say, living with the wrong shade of wallpaper.

ACUPRESSURE

The main development out of acupuncture has been 'acupressure', developed as 'schiatsu' in Japan in the eighteenth century. It remained in relative obscurity there until about fifty years ago when it began to become fashionable, partly because it dispensed with needles, but also because it did not have to be as accurately directed as in traditional acupuncture, so that it could be relatively easily learned in the family. The pressure is usually applied with the knuckles, or the ball of the thumb, the end-product often being described as a cross between acupuncture and massage, and its effect as being between pleasure and pain. When it was tried out recently in a hospital for autistic children in Oakland, California, the results astonished the researchers. The children's reaction was often emotionally as well as physically explosive, 'a release of physical and emotional energy'; but their initial displays of anger and fear were followed by a catharsis, restoring the therapist to 'a gentle and loving communication from the child'.

MANIPULATION

Of the alternative therapies based on the use of manipulation and massage, the 'Alexander Principle' can lay claim to the most illustrious list of supporters. Around the end of the last century F. Matthias Alexander, an Australian, came to the conclusion that although the osteopaths were right in their contention that a great many diverse symptoms could be traced to the spine, it was not maladjustment of the vertebrae which was responsible but faulty posture. Habit, he decided, affects use; and use affects function. If people habitually misuse their bodies by adopting postures for which they are not designed they cannot expect their muscular or nervous systems to function satisfactorily.

What appears to come naturally to us, Alexander insisted, is not necessarily right for us. It may represent the result of a protracted period of misuse, which can only be corrected by following a course of exercises designed to restore conscious control of all movements. To do this the patient must be constantly on the watch for subconscious processes which have led to the faulty movements, and always have in mind the correct movements with which to replace them, so that he can deliberately perform them until they come naturally and subconsciously.

Like most such techniques, though, it is impossible to describe satisfactorily (as Alexander replied when taxed with his own inability to put it across in his books, nobody expects to learn golf from a manual of instruction). But among those who testified to its effectiveness have been John Dewey, Bernard Shaw, Sir Charles Sherrington and Aldous Huxley. 'It gives us all the things we have been looking for in a system of medical education,' Huxley wrote in his *Ends and Means*, 'relief from strain due to maladjustment and consequent improvement in mental and physical health.'

Receiving the Nobel Prize for Physiology and Medicine in 1974, Nikolaas Tinbergen, Professor of Animal Behaviour at Oxford University, remarked that he and his fellow award-winners, Lorenz and von Frisch, had been honoured for following the ancient method of 'watching and wondering'; and this, he recalled, was the method Alexander had used. Blinded by the glamour of laboratory apparatus, scientists now tend to look down on it, and the medical profession has largely ignored the Alexander Principle – a mistake, Tinbergen feels, as it 'is an extremely sophisticated form of rehabilitation, or rather of redeployment, of the entire muscular equipment, and through that of many other organs'; compared to it 'many other common types of physiotherapy look crude'.

One of the other common types, 'Rolfing', certainly looks – and feels – crude. In the 1940's Ida Rolf, then a research chemist at the Rockefeller Institute, decided to take up Hatha Yoga; and in trying it out she came to the conclusion that what she and most other people needed was a preliminary course of structural re-integration. Like Alexander, she felt that bad postural habits needed to be broken down; but she did not believe that there had to be elaborate re-training. By analogy, she argued, the human body is like a child's tower of bricks. If they are not aligned correctly on top of each other, the whole structure wobbles. The muscles are consequently kept so occupied holding it upright that they cannot easily perform their proper functions; they lose their elasticity, and adhesions form, imprisoning bones and muscles. What is required, she decided, is a short, sharp course in which the body is kneaded, pummeled and jabbed, in a painful in-depth form of massage, designed to break down the adhesions so as to liberate bones, ligaments and muscles to work freely again with the bricks back in their correct alignment. Having once enjoyed the experience which this freedom gives the Rolfed individual will be careful not to lose it, all the more so because he knows the agonies he will have to endure if he has to go through the procedure again; and he will enjoy freedom not only from backache, arthritis and other such disorders, but also a general improvement of health. Since the 1960s Ida Rolf has been training students to carry on her work; her disciples and imitators are beginning to establish themselves in Britain and in other European countries, as well as throughout Northern America.

A relatively new development in this manipulation category is 'applied kinesiology': the application ordinarily being by members of the 'Touch for Health' movement. Their idea is that it is possible to detect weakness and incipient disease in the organs of the body before symptoms actually appear, simply by the 'feel' of certain muscles. It is primarily a diagnostic technique, therefore, and is commonly used in conjunction with chiropractic. Other manipulative methods include 'cranial osteopathy', manipulation of the skull; and 'reflexology', based on the assumption that there is a connection between the nerve endings in the feet and the organs of the body, so that on much the same principle as applied kinesiology, anything which is wrong with the organs can be detected. It can also, by the appropriate form of foot massage, be treated. Some practitioners insist that the procedure is mechanical; heat, say, or swellings, provide them with clues. Others use a method more resembling braille, as if they were acquiring diagnostic information not simply by touch but also by some sixth sense. Treatment varies according to the ideas and experience of the therapist; but it ranges between stroking and massage.

PSYCHIC HEALERS

The fourth category of traditional therapies consists of those close to tribal shamanism. Although they have yet to make much headway in Europe or North America, except in a few religious sects, they have made an impact through books, articles and TV programmes and the controversies they have often aroused. They have important implications, too, for medicine because even more forcibly than spiritual healing or radiesthesia they present a challenge to orthodox assumptions. If what has been reported about psychic healers in Brazil and in the Philippines could be convincingly demonstrated to the satisfaction (or, in this case, intense dissatisfaction) of orthodox medical scientists, it would not necessarily bring about any revolutionary changes in Western clinical practice, any more than acupuncture has been able to do, because the transmission, or graft, might not 'take'. But it would certainly provide an explanation for much that has been considered inexplicable in history, and for some cures which in recent times have been greeted as miraculous by the faithful, and derided by sceptics as fakes.

The first of the shaman healers to attract attention outside his home country, Brazil, was 'Arigo'. Born in 1921, Arigo had little formal education and no medical training; but he became a healer in the shaman tradition that still flourished in the country, reinvigorated by an infusion of spiritism deriving from the influence of Allan Kardec, the nineteenth century psychic whose teachings found a more receptive public there than they did in Europe.

Arigo claimed no healing powers for himself, believing that he was taken over by 'Dr Fritz', a deceased German, who told him what was the matter with patients, and if necessary performed surgical operations on them, using Arigo as his human medium. He would treat as many as three hundred patients every day. As they came to him, in turn, he would make an almost instantaneous diagnosis. According to Andrija Puharich, who went twice to test him in the 1960s and checked on about a thousand of his findings, not merely was Arigo astonishingly accurate but he often used the correct medical terminology. Puharich, himself a doctor, asked him how he did it. 'I simply listen to a voice in my right ear,' Arigo told him, 'and repeat what it says.'

Having made his diagnosis, Arigo would prescribe; and the medicine he recommended might be a pharmacological compound of a kind which he could not have been expected to know about – a drug just marketed in Europe, for example – which Puharich would find on enquiry was appropriate. Even more disconcerting, though, was his surgery. Arigo would pull out an unsterilised pocket knife, or use a knife from the kitchen, to open up patients' bodies. He had no need for sutures or stitches, because he could halt the flow of blood by a word of command. There was no post-operative infection; the wounds healed much more rapidly than such wounds ordinarily do, sometimes instantaneously; and patients felt little or no pain.

Coming as they did from Puharich – a senior research scientist at the New York University Medical Center, and Director of Research of an American Corporation – these reports carried weight; but his later involvement with parapsychology, and in particular the fact that he became Uri Geller's mentor, subsequently lessened his credibility. As always when a new recruit joins the ranks of those who accept paranormal phenomena, it is a signal for sceptics to belittle the value of his earlier research on the ground that he has since revealed his gullibility. But his evidence has been confirmed by several later investigators; notably by Guy Playfair, who has described his researches into Kardeckian spiritism and other psychical phenomena in the eccentrically titled but serious study, *The Flying Cow*; and by Arigo's American biographer, John G. Fuller. And among those who were convinced of Arigo's powers by personal experience, sometimes actually on the operating table, were several doctors, including Juscelino Kubitschek, President of Brazil, who had trained as a surgeon at the Sorbonne.

Ordinarily the Brazilian authorities, though they mistrust spiritism, have left the healers alone, knowing how popular they are. Arigo, though, became too popular and he was arrested for illegally practising medicine. An even more striking testimonial to him than the accounts which had been published of his cures (and films showing him at work) was the fact that no patient appeared to testify against him. Ironically, as Fuller observed, it was what grateful patients were saying in his favour that made his conviction on the charge inevitable; and although on the first occasion he was released on the President's intervention, when Kubitschek was no longer in office Arigo was again arrested, and spent seven months in jail.

For Arigo imprisonment was not the shattering experience it had been for Reich or Drown. It gave him the first rest, he realised, that he had enjoyed for years; and the publicity established his reputation nationally. He hoped that this would persuade the medical profession to take his claims seriously, and a few doctors, including sceptics, who came to watch him went away convinced that he was genuine. He was never detected in any trickery. But no formal invitation came to him to demonstrate his method at a medical research institute, in Brazil or elsewhere. In 1971 he told Kubitschek he had had a premonition that he was soon to die a violent death. A few weeks later he was killed in a road-crash.

Scores of other healers practise in Brazil along similar lines; some, like Lourival de Freitas, even more unconventional in their methods. His preparation for work consists of guitar-playing, accompanied by draughts of Scotch whisky; but his record of cures cannot easily be discounted. Such performers disturb Spiritualists even more than they annoy sceptics. As the British healer Gordon Turner put it, if it is spirit healing why the need for a knife? And even where shaman-type healers do not use knives, as in the Philippines, Spiritualists are uneasy. Some argue that the spirits understandably use any human instrument that serves their purposes; but others share the sceptics' view that the whole procedure must be a squalid racket.

In *Wonder Healers of the Philippines,* published in 1968, the American psychical researcher Harold Sherman described the work of some of the Philippine healers, notably Tony Agpaoa. At the age of nine Agpaoa had a spiritual experience of the kind which in tribal communities traditionally identifies the shaman-to-be; he appeared to be possessed, taken over by his 'protector' – guardian angel, or daemon, or spirit guide – who instructed him that he was to be a healer. He had no need for a knife; Sherman watched him knead patients' stomachs until blood began to come through, and the flesh to part: out would come the tumour; the flesh would be rolled back again; and – apparently instantaneously – the stomach would heal, leaving no trace of the operation, not so much as a hair-line scar.

At the same time as Sherman was investigating a few entrepreneurs were waking up to the possibility of laying on package tours to bring rich Americans to the Philippines for treatment. Inevitably this traffic has spawned bogus practitioners, and doubtless corrupted some genuine healers; and there have been several cases where sleight-of-hand has been alleged. In 1975 a producer from a British television company managed to snatch a 'tumour' which had just been removed from a patient's stomach; laboratory analysis revealed that it came from a farmyard animal. In the same year Judge Daniel H. Hanscom delivered his verdict in an action brought by the Federal Trade Commission against the travel agencies who had run the tours; on the evidence, he had decided, psychic surgery was 'pure and unmitigated fakery'.

The evidence, though, as Krippner and Villoldo have shown in *The Realms of Psychic Healing*, is not so damning as it has been made to appear. The motives of some of the witnesses who have provided it are suspect: either they went to the Philippines with their minds already made up, or they were aware that a de-bunking exercise would be profitable. The judge in his summing-up, too, simply ignored testimony favourable to psychic surgery, such as that of the Californian biologist, Donald Westerbeke, who after a careful survey had concluded that although many healers resorted to sleight-of-hand some of the time, and a few all the time, some were genuine.

But even if sleight-of-hand has been employed, this is not necessarily proof of fraudulent intent. What many of the commentators have not realised is that psychic surgery is neither confined to the Philippines nor, as William Nolen claimed it was in his *Healing: a doctor in search of a miracle*, a recent development. So commonly did psychic surgery feature in the reports of tribal communities in the mid-nineteenth century that Edward Tylor felt compelled to admit in his *Primitive Culture* that he was disturbed by the implications. He could not account for it rationally, except on the presumption of sleight-of-hand. But neither could he accept that all witch doctors and medicine men who practised it were cheats.

If they were not cheats, there were two possible explanations: that the shamans had psychokinetic powers, or that the procedure was symbolic. The belief that illness is caused by spirits or sorcerers insinuating a pebble into the body of their victims could be found even in advanced societies like the Aztecs, Rivers noted in his *Medicine, Magic and Religion*, published in 1924; and this suggested that even if the object 'sucked out' by the shaman were an ordinary pebble, it could still be held to have a legitimate therapeutic function. In such cases, if the shaman is aware that it is the suggestion of sorcery which is responsible for the symptoms, 'the sight of the offending object thus said to have been removed effects a rapid cure in removing the suggestion'.

In his *History of Medicine* Sigerist took this argument a step further. Like Tylor, he could not believe that shamans had fooled their people with such cheap tricks. The explanation, he felt, was that as the offending object was assumed to have been introduced into the patient's body 'not physically but magically', it would be taken for granted that it must be removed in the same way. The pebble in the shaman's mouth, then, might be regarded as a fetish: an object charged with psychic power, kept for that purpose. 'By performing the rites, of which sucking is one, he expects his object to attract the foreign body from the patient's parts so that the two become one magically. Thus he can produce the object with all sincerity'.

Evidence has since accumulated to suggest these explanations are correct. Anthropological field workers have reported being assured that, though an object may be 'pouched', there is no fraudulent intent. Working in the Achumawi community in the 1920s, Jaime de Angulo was told by one of them that the shaman always had the object which he was going to extract in his mouth before the operation. 'But he draws the sickness into them, he uses them to catch the poison. Otherwise how could he catch it?' In Africa in the 1960s some diviners admitted to John Beattie that they only pretended to draw the objects out of patients. They insisted, though that this did not mean they were cheating. They believed they could 'hold' or 'seize' the sickness in the object, 'and that was the most important aspect of the whole process'.

The nearest parallel in the Western world is the doctrine of transubstantiation; snatching a 'tumour' from a psychic surgeon for laboratory analysis is, in fact, hardly more sensible than snatching communion bread and wine from a priest for the same 'scientific' purpose. The fact that the objects extracted now tend to resemble human gut and tissue is not necessarily proof of fraud; the more likely explanation is that as communities become more sophisticated, in Western terms, their members cease to believe in the ability of a sorcerer to insinuate pebbles into the bodies of his victims, and accept that he makes them ill by starting up disease processes within the body.

Even if psychic surgeons in the Philippines do not really have psychic powers, this does not mean that they necessarily stand condemned. But there is evidence that some of them, at least, do have paranormal powers. It is not easy to dispute the testimony of scores of people who have themselves been operated upon, and watched the whole procedure (among them Peter Sellers, who has described how healers made incisions just by touching him, and then probed around inside his body, painlessly, while he was watching, and while his wife was taking photographs). There have also been a few carefully-conducted investigations. In 1973 a team of nine scientists, doctors, physicists and psychiatrists, led by George Meek, brought fifty patients to the Philippines for treatment by ten healers. In their report they unanimously agreed that there had been no fraud, and that although there had been no precautions against sepsis, there had been no infections. Some of the patients, too – including one of the investigators – were cured of what had been considered inoperable conditions.

Individual observers have also reported phenomena which, they feel, cannot be accounted for by sleight-of-hand. In *The Romeo Error* Lyall Watson has described how he watched Juan Blance of Pasig make incisions by simply pointing his finger, a variant of the shaman's 'pointing the bone'. The cut could be made in this way even when Watson placed a plastic sheet between Blance's finger and the patient. Krippner had a similar experience: about to treat a patient who was lying on her stomach, Blance indicated to him that he should extend the finger of his right hand; then took Krippner's right hand and directed his forefinger at the woman's back, about six inches away from it. 'Suddenly he made an abrupt motion with my forefinger, then released it,' Krippner – himself an amateur magician – recalls. 'I noticed a slit on the woman's skin in the exact area beneath my finger position. Within a few seconds, a thin ribbon of blood filled this slit.'

Another phenomenon reported by some investigators, Watson among them, is the de-materialisation of objects which they have collected after psychic surgery demonstrations. In Watson's case, he had taken away a specimen for analysis; the following morning the jar in which he had put it was empty, though the seal was still intact. And this raises what is increasingly coming to be accepted as the fundamental problem in psycho-psychics. *If* objects can materialise and de-materialise, as psychical researchers (and families plagued by a poltergeist) have so often reported, then normal precautions against fraud become inadequate.

If a shaman were capable of materialising objects in his patients' bodies, he would presumably wish the objects to appear in the form patients expected them to appear. In tribal communities, for some reason, pebbles and thorns seem to have been the common expectation. In medieval times 'nails and hair, needles, bristles, pieces of glass and many other things have been pulled out of the bodies of patients while the physicians stood by helpless,' Paracelsus noted. 'Had they understood their business, they would have known that these things had been brought into the body by the power of the evil imagination of a sorcerer.' If, in the Philippines, patients expect blood or tissue or tumours, and the healer has the required psychic powers, he naturally materialises substances which look human. But as he would not have needed to ensure they were 'real' – not, at least, until investigators began to arrive who would have them tested in laboratories – he would have no need to materialise human blood, or tissue or tumours; though he might himself believe that this was what he was doing.

REINCARNATION –
EXORCISM – ASTROLOGY

Psychic healing is hard to treat dispassionately, because to accept it as a valid and potentially valuable form of treatment involves accepting the existence of forces of a kind which are still unacceptable to orthodox medical science, and alien to common experience (and often, common sense). But there are a few aspirants to public recognition in this category which would also until very recently have been dismissed out of hand in Western countries, but which have now begun to achieve a measure of credibility.

One is reincarnation, in which there has been a marked revival of interest, partly through greater familiarity with the 'karma' tradition, partly because of the evidence from the meticulous research of Professor Ian Stevenson of the University of Virginia, and from tape recordings of hypnotised subjects who have been 'regressed' to past lives – notably those made in Cardiff by Arnall Bloxham, presented on a BBC television programme and later analysed in *More Lives than One?* by the producer, Jeffrey Iverson. There is now a 'past lives therapy'; and Arthur Guirdham has been arguing persuasively in his books that it is necessary to bear the possibility of such psychic intrusion in mind, not only in treating psychiatric disorders which can be caused, he believes, by people misinterpreting the information which comes through from a discarnate self (the recipients may fear that they are suffering from incipient insanity); but also in diagnosing physical ailments some of which, in his experience, represent a kind of replay of traumatic episodes from a past life.

Exorcism has also been returning to acceptance, if not as yet to favour, among both Catholic and Protestant churchmen. It presents something of a problem, particularly to Protestants, as belief in the devil has been eroded. Still, it is possible to think in terms of generalised forces of evil manifesting themselves in particular (and sometimes personal) forms which, being psychic in nature, need psychic or spiritual shock treatment. And exorcism provides the clergy with a therapeutic device which they can use to re-establish their long neglected healing mission. The reaction of individuals to exorcism, however, is notoriously unpredictable, and although the convulsions so often associated with it can be regarded – as they were by shamans, and later by Mesmer – as an indication that the treatment is working, or as a sign that the forces of evil are being expelled, they can be alarming to watch, and hard to control.

A third contender for recognition as a therapeutic aid is astrology. In his tests of psychic diagnosticians Shealy also tried out an astrologer, who was correct with one third of his patients: not so high a proportion as the psychics obtained, but significantly above chance expectation. And some therapists have begun to use it, as Jung did, to provide an additional guide both in diagnosis and in deciding upon treatment. As Liz Greene has argued in *Relating*, it is not yet known whether there is any material basis for the correlation of astrological data with human behaviour; 'but Michael Gauquelin's laborious and thorough statistical research has demonstrated that such correlations are valid'; and if valid, they have some relevance to the practice of medicine.

THE GROWTH MOVEMENT

Most forms of traditional medicine, then, are expanding. And the late developer, psychotherapy (the term only came into use a century ago), has already become the most diversified of all; the hardest, too, to summarise, not simply because of the diversity but also because it does not fit the general pattern.

In physical medicine the distinction between orthodox and unorthodox is fairly clear; in psychotherapy it is confused. On the organisational level distinctions can be made. Some groups are accredited within the health services, others are not – though they may be seeking recognition: a National Council of Psychotherapists was formed in Britain in the early 1970s when individuals in practice round the country realised that their right to continue to give treatment was threatened by a report from Sir John Foster, QC, urging legislation to restrict it to members of approved bodies. But most psychotherapists are either doctors, lay analysts trained by doctors, clinical psychologists or psychiatric social workers. They do not consider themselves as paramedical, even if the methods they use are regarded by orthodox psychiatrists as unconventional, and by their colleagues in the medical profession as eccentric.

Nevertheless unconventional psychotherapy (as it may for convenience be called) has arisen largely because of a growing conviction that, in Carl Rogers' words, 'The medical model is an extremely inappropriate one for dealing with psychological disturbances.' How inappropriate it has become was to some extent disguised by two developments in conventional phychiatry during the past half-century. One was the recognition that whatever may be the contributory causes of mental breakdown – genetic, constitutional, environmental or biochemical – the symptoms of psychosis were in fact largely the consequence of locking people up in lunatic asylums and leaving them there without hope of release. The 'open door' system, introduced by a few courageous psychiatrists in the 1940s, revealed that simply liberating patients from such incarceration cured quite a high proportion of them, at least temporarily.

The second development was the introduction of new forms of treatment: tranquillisers and anti-depressants, electroconvulsive therapy, and leucotomy – brain operations. For a while these lulled psychiatrists into a belief that they had found at least a partial solution to the problem of mental illness. But during the last two decades it has become unhappily apparent (though not to all psychiatrists) that leucotomies have been discredited; that ECT's value is unproven; and that together with psychotropic drugs they have replaced the 'open door' with (as somebody put it) the 'revolving door', because so many patients need to return to mental hospitals for further treatment. And the rapidly increasing number of prescriptions for psychotropic drugs for patients outside mental hospitals is causing serious concern.

What unconventional psychotherapy is offering, according to Rogers, is 'a potential for growth and development, that can be released in the right psychological climate'. The 'growth movement', as it has come to be known, reflects dissatisfaction not just with conventional psychiatry, but with the whole idea that mental illness can be treated by pills and operations. It takes a bewildering variety of forms, many of them having their origins in Freudian theory. And of these, the first to attract attention, and sometimes notoriety, were the 'encounter groups' which began to form in the early 1960s.

Group therapy had originally been a device by which psycho-analysts tried to get round the problem of having more patients than they could handle one by one; but it was found that some patients appeared to do better in a group setting, and as adopted and then extended by Rogers in Chicago, the method enabled people to shed their inhibitions in circumstances where they could be sure of supportive company. Ordinarily, though, 'encounter' in this context has referred to groups in which displays of repressed emotion are not simply allowed, but are deliberately induced by the therapist or members of the group. Patients may be told to insult each other until one of them loses control, the collapse into tears or rage being regarded as the first step in what might be called the Rolfing of the personality, to liberate the true psyche by breaking down society's adhesions.

A variant of encounter therapy is 'psychodrama'. It can trace its roots back to tribal medicine, where a similar technique has often been recorded by anthropologists as in use in the treatment of mental illness. Participants are given dramatic roles to act out, in the expectation that they will give clues to hidden or repressed feelings; as Claudius did when he saw the Player King re-enact the murder of Hamlet's father (though in modern psychodrama it it usually the actors whose emotional response is being monitored).

The most striking development of the encounter principle, though, has been 'est' – Erhard Seminars Training, founded by Werner Erhard in 1971. In each training session, two hundred and fifty people come together for two consecutive weekends in a hotel ballroom, and sit on uncomfortable chairs during four twelve-hour sessions without eating, drinking, smoking or pill-taking. Originally there was only one break in the middle of each session (in New York, Adelaide Bry recalls in her book on est, it was called the 'no piss training' because no trainee was permitted to leave the room in the course of a session – or, rather, anybody who left was not permitted to return). Now, there are breaks every four hours; but otherwise the method is the same. The two hundred and fifty trainees are confronted by their trainer, who leads off by telling them that they are all 'assholes'; they are machines, little more than tubes through which food and drink run in a neverending stream. But they must have grasped that something is the matter, or they would not be at the seminar. 'You people are here today because all of your strategies, your smart-ass theories, and all the rest of your shit hasn't worked for you,' Bry heard her trainer say. 'All of your fucking cleverness and self-deception have gotten you nowhere.'

The aim, as in other encounter groups, is to induce resentment, frustration, rage; but est often does more. The effects can resemble those described in accounts of Mesmer's sessions, and of shamanism: the trainees lose control, with shudderings, nausea, vomiting and other symptoms ordinarily associated with hysteria. Some individuals emerge appalled by what they have been brought through; others – a high enough proportion to have made est an extremely profitable organisation, at the (1975) fee of $200 (£100) for a course – are so impressed that their enthusiasm has continued to infect friends and acquaintances with the desire to go through the training, in spite of the prospect of the abuse and the hysterics.

The various forms of 'primal therapy' come in this category, derived as they are from Freud's discovery that a child, when not allowed to show feelings, builds defences to disguise hurt, and that these develop into neuroses. But the protagonist of the best-known version, Janov, insists that the unconscious is 'real and healthy', and that it is simply the defences that make us 'unreal and maladapted'. His cure is to help patients regress to infancy, the 'primal scream' providing them with the first intimation that long-bottled-up tensions are being released. Primal therapy, Janov insists, is not just another version of psychotherapy; not merely does it purport 'to *cure* mental illness (psycho-physical illness to be exact)', but 'it claims to be the only cure'. 'It', in this case, is presumably shorthand for 'its founder'; Janov is not troubled by false modesty.

The same principle has been quite widely adopted in the

rather different form of encouraging people to give vent to their feelings by screaming, or yelling – where it is practicable to do so: Bricklin in his *Encyclopedia of Natural Healing* advocates 'inner shouting' on the ground that 'if you do it out loud you might be carted away'. The therapeutic value, Bricklin claims, lies in the fact that the shouters focus their attention on the hurts and pains, rather than on anger and frustration, and this helps them to analyse the true cause of their feelings.

In his *Gestalt Therapy*, Fritz Perls also emphasised the closeness of the links between suppressed emotions and physical ailments. Children's inclination to yell their heads off when thwarted, he argued, could lead, if parents or teachers blocked it, to faulty posture; and that in turn could promote backache, or headaches in later life. The cure is not to go to the doctor for pills, but to learn how to release tensions. But at this point his thesis diverges from Janov's. Gestalt therapy consists of throwing off inhibitions and adopting the existentialist attitude of 'humanistic hedonism' – a determination to enjoy the present to the full, though at the same time realising that such enjoyment is not to be confused with self-indulgence.

Like Janov, Eric Berne lost confidence in Freudian analysis; and in the 1950s he began to develop his own 'transactional analysis', basically a way of speeding up the analytic process of observing and learning how to deal with the ruses and rationalisations which hold it back: the 'games people play'. The games, Berne found, are also played in organisations, such as business firms; thus incidentally confirming the findings of research by the Tavistock Centre in London undertaken with groups of executives, which has revealed how necessary it is to take job-dissatisfaction into account as one of the causes of ill-health.

In *Psychosynthesis*, published in 1965, Roberto Assagioli offered another variation. Intuition, he complained, has been repressed 'by non-recognition, devaluation, neglect and lack of connection with other psychological functions'; by cultivating it individuals can tap 'a precious function which generally remains latent and unused'.

These and other sources, Jungian as well as Freudian, have

given birth to the Humanistic Psychology Association formed by Rogers, Perls, Maslow and others to promote what Maslow called 'high-level wellness' – health a grade above the ordinary conception, absence of disease. Humanistic Psychology is not so much psychotherapy in its own right as a reflection of the need to provide a synthesis of existing therapies; the Association's aim is to promote their use 'as a means of developing awareness and sensitivity' in the hope that they will help to 'build a society in which people are valued as creative self-realising persons'.

It is not only unconventional psychotherapies, though, which have contributed to the development of the growth movement. It has also been loosely linked with cults: the successors of Madame Blavatsky's Theosophy, Steiner's Anthroposophy, and Gurdjieff's 'fourth way'. Some of them in fact began *as* psychotherapies: when Ron Hubbard's *Dianetics: the modern science of mental health* was published in 1950 it presented Scientology as a counterblast to orthodox psychiatry. Within five years, however, the opening of a 'Church of Scientology' in Washington showed the way the movement was going; and although it kept up its campaigns against orthodox psychiatry – particularly in Britain, where Hubbard established the movement's headquarters – its sectarian element, demanding loyalty, prevented Scientology from becoming a serious alternative. Its management's attempts to silence criticism by litigation proved an expensive failure, alienating many people who would otherwise have been sympathetic; and an ill-conceived attempt to take over the Establishment body, the National Association for Mental Health, simply provoked government reprisals. Scientology has now backed away from controversy: it describes itself as a 'religious philosophy containing pastoral procedures, aiming to provide spiritual freedom'. It has thereby extricated itself from a process which has had destructive consequences for other ventures, initially as well-intentioned, Synanon for example.

Synanon was founded in California by Charles Dederich in 1958 as a psychotherapy centre offering 'psychic restructuring', a form of encounter therapy designed to give patients, and in particular hard drug addicts, the self-reliance they needed to be able to regulate their lives. So encouraging were the early reports that the Synanon system was adopted in many States during the 1960s, until it was found that although the inmates could keep off heroin so long as they remained within the system, it did little or nothing to improve their chances of staying off heroin when they left. By this time, however, Synanon had attracted a cult following. Defiantly, Dederich persuaded the faithful to demonstrate their solidarity with him by shaving their heads, and even swopping wives; and at the same time he started libel suits for over a hundred million dollars against newspapers which had carried articles criticising the physical violence into which encounter therapy had sometimes degenerated. In 1978 Dederich was arrested, accused of soliciting two members of his sect, as by this time it had become, to put a rattlesnake (with the rattle removed, to ensure that it would give no warning) into the postbox of one of the lawyers who had appeared against him; and the court hearing had to be postponed because the magistrate decided that, on the evidence, Dederich was of unsound mind.

Dederich's arrest happened to coincide with the news of the enforced mass suicide of the members of the Rev. Jim Jones' Peoples' Temple in Guyana, another warning of the risks run by any project designed to break down personality defences. The avowed aim may be to allow the individual to rebuild them along his own lines; but lacking them, he is tempted to let them be rebuilt for him along lines which his guru or his commune happen to favour. Cults tend to corrupt; absolutist cults corrupt absolutely.

AUTO-SUGGESTION – YOGA

Of all the contributors to the growth movement, potentially the most influential is the consequence of the coming together of auto-suggestion, on the Coué/Schultz model, with yoga, a union in which biofeedback was the catalyst.

Coué-style auto-suggestion was revived as a therapy in the United States by José Silva. Experimenting with hypnotism,

Silva found that instructing subjects how to hypnotise themselves into keeping well was more effective; and in the 1950s he developed his 'mind control' method which, his organisation claims, has since been enthusiastically endorsed by over half a million people ranging from Hollywood stars to the Chicago White Sox baseball team. At the same time, Wolfgang Luthe of Montreal was instructing patients how to practise Schultz's autogenic training. The link was forged by Elmer Green and his wife, when they invited the Indian Swami Rama for tests at the Menninger Foundation. They found that he was able to regulate the flow of blood so that there was a difference of as much as five degrees centigrade between his two hands. When he said he would show the Greens that he could stop his heart from beating the recorded tape appeared to show that on the contrary, it rose from seventy to three hundred beats a minute, for a period of seventeen seconds. A cardiologist, however, told the Greens that this must have been 'flutter' of a kind which happens only when the heart is *not* functioning as a pump. Normally, when this occurs, the patient faints. Swami Rama 'just took off the electrodes and went out and gave a lecture'.

The claims made on behalf of yogi had attracted some attention from psychical researchers, but little notice in the medical profession, even after the Maharishi had visited Europe and America to popularise transcendental meditation. But Green's evidence could not be attributed to fakir-style trickery, and it quickly became apparent that anybody and everybody had some ability of the kind, which could be developed with the help of auto-suggestion and biofeedback. In the experimental stages this lead to a remarkable re-approachment between two old irreconcilables, the behaviourists and the analytically-orientated psychologists. Biofeedback had originally been developed by behaviourists Neal Miller and Herbert Benson; but the evidence derived from it provided massive justification for the psychosomatic theories put forward a quarter of a century before, chiefly by Freudians. And the validity of Selye's stress theory was even more convincingly demonstrated.

It took time, though, for the implications to seep through to the medical profession. In the mid-1970s most people who wanted to try auto-suggestion had to seek it in one of the many organisations offering yoga. Biofeedback machines, too, were more commonly recommended as part of the training in such groups than they were by doctors; particularly in Britain, where until the late 1970s it was unusual to find even one such machine in any hospital. Recently a few reports of trials showing the effectiveness of meditation as a replacement for psychotropic drugs have been beginning to appear in the medical journals; and in 1978 a group of doctors formally petitioned the Minister of Health urging that transcendental meditation should be made available on the National Health Service. But so far as the public is concerned meditation and biofeedback are still regarded as unconventional forms of treatment. Certainly few people go to their GPs and ask for them. And most of the important experimental work, such as that which is being carried out in Britain by Maxwell Cade, has received little notice and less support from the medical Establishment.

One of Cade's experiments, in conjunction with Ann Woolley-Hart, has helped to answer what has long been a puzzling question: why hypnotherapy, which so often over the past two centuries has given satisfactory and sometimes spectacular results, has never succeeded in establishing itself. They gave one group of twenty volunteers instruction in psychosomatics, coupled with group hypnotherapy, while another group received the same instructions, but with relaxation and autogenic exercises instead of the hypnotherapy. The therapeutic effect was much more impressive, they found, with the second group. Suggestion, it appears, can be a useful therapeutic aid, especially when reinforced by hypnosis; but the effect is relatively superficial. It seems unlikely, therefore, that hypnotism will stage yet another of its periodic comebacks. Yet it could still find a place as an adjunct to autogenic training and to healing – as it was for Edgar Cayce. The pattern emerging from Cade's research, and from Shealy's, is of a fusion of hypnotic suggestion, auto-suggestion, relaxation, biofeedback and healing, supplementing and complementing each other.

CROSS-FERTILISATION

It is no longer possible, then, to think in terms of expanding existing health services simply by inviting the main alternative therapies to set their houses in order, and present themselves for a vetting process to decide whether they are suitable for admission. The process of fission has gone too far. But there is another and probably even more important reason why any system designed to give, say, qualified manipulators or acupuncturists statutory recognition would now be unwise. Alternative medicine is in a state of flux, rendering some traditional groupings obsolescent.

'In the past decade,' Denis T. Jaffe observed in his *In Search of a Therapy*, published in 1975, psychotherapy 'has broadened from the traditional activities of physician-psychiatrist and clinical psychologist to include many new forms and styles, often practised by people who do not have the usual credentials or training'. The therapist, therefore, 'can no longer learn a skill in a professional school and then practice it, with a few modifications, for the rest of his or her life' – a view confirmed by a number of the contributors to his book, describing what they had been taught, and how they had been led to try very different methods. And the process seems likely to accelerate, as more and more practitioners realise the benefits of combining psychotherapy with other forms of treatment.

The method which has attracted the most attention has been developed by Carl Simonton, a radiologist from Fort Worth in Texas, who has introduced a novel form of Couéism, 'visualisation therapy', encouraging cancer patients to conjure up a mental picture of themselves fighting the growths with the help of any analogy – a battlefield, say – that may stimulate the imagination. In Britain Ian Pearce, a general practitioner, has been working on similar lines, using meditation to assist the process; the patient is directed 'to turn his eyes within and to try to see *his* disease, to visualise his pain, his disordered function, and then, while looking at the disease, to visualise the cells of the body attacking, surrounding and confining his disease, and finally destroying it'.

The possibility of linking psychotherapy with psychic healing has also attracted researchers on both sides of the Atlantic: Lawrence LeShan in New York, and Ann Woolley-Hart in London. Her experiments have followed an unsuccessful attempt by Harry Edwards shortly before his death to persuade the medical profession to investigate his healing. A committee was set up under McCausland's chairmanship which, as a preliminary, tried to circulate a questionnaire to cancer victims; but the Cancer Foundations, with their unspent millions, looked the other way, and the national newspapers refused to print advertisements asking for people to fill in the questionnaire, so the project fell through. In its place, Woolley-Hart – a doctor who had herself been operated on for cancer – and a healer, Gilbert Anderson, set up a pilot project, combining psychotherapy on a group and individual basis, with meditation and healing. After nineteen months of regular meetings, four out of the five patients were found on medical examination to have no apparent traces of cancer; but as trials of this kind take at least five years before even a preliminary assessment of the results is considered permissible, and as the project is on so small a scale, it will require other projects of a more elaborate kind if such methods are to engage the medical profession's attention.

Cross-fertilisation has also begun to exert a powerful influence on other branches of traditional medicine, notably on manipulative treatment.

The pioneer of what might be described as psycho-manipulation, though he calls it bioenergetics, has been Alexander Lowen, one of Reich's students. In his *Physical Dynamics of Character Structure*, published in 1958, Lowen presented his case that where orthodox psycho-analysis was inadequate was in its failure to recognise the need to release physical as well as emotional tension; it is necessary, he argued, to learn 'the language of the body' (the title under which the book reached a wider audience in paper-back) as well as of the unconscious mind. And he has since built up a physiological counterpart to psycho-analysis. 'Lacking a fair grounding in the body,' he wrote in 1976, 'the ego has no feeling of reality'; as a result, its knowledge degenerates into abstractions, whereas 'contact with the body provides the ego with an understanding of internal reality'. Bioenergetics is designed to improve mind-body inter-relationship by emphasising the importance of, for example, a good stance ('feet on the ground'), and good breathing habits.

As it happens, Lowen's ideas are not far removed from those of F. M. Alexander. Delivering a memorial lecture in his memory, Marjorie Barlow has emphasised that Alexander felt that 'postural' was too narrow a term to describe his therapy, because bad posture is 'misuse of the self', the end result of psychological as well as physical processes. Ida Rolf, too, evolved her techniques from Hatha Yoga when she found its teachers were expert 'in refining the body for the express purpose of furthering individual psychic expression'. Some of her followers have taken up this idea; one of the contributors to Jaffe's *In Search of a Therapy*, Don Johnson, described how during his training as a Jesuit priest he was not allowed to touch any other Jesuit, except in formal greeting. But progressive Catholics welcomed some aspects of encounter therapy; he decided to participate in an encounter group, and what he experienced led him to leave the Jesuits and enrol under Rolf. In his experience, 'when the hands of the Rolfer (or elbow, or knuckle) release the hang-ups of the flesh, the ego is partially broken'; Rolfing is consequently a political, or metapolitical, activity, which involves 'a new discipline, consonant with a new way of seeing'.

At the same time, some osteopaths have been becoming aware of the implications of acupuncture and of acupressure; a school of 'osteopuncture' has been founded in California. Others have been tempted to move still further from tradi-tional techniques. What has happened has been described by Harold Klug, a lecturer at the European School of Osteopathy and editor of the *Journal of the Society of Osteopaths*. Dis-cussing among themselves what methods were the most effec-tive, some osteopaths admitted they were drawn to the idea of encouraging muscles and ligaments to unwind, rather than giving a twist or thrust to break down adhesions. It was the patient, after all, whose reaction had tensed the muscles: what would happen if the osteopath's hands were placed on the patient, with no attempt to massage or manipulate? The answer was that sometimes the ligaments and muscles holding the joint appeared to relax, as it were, of their own accord. As one of the American osteopaths who developed the system, Vera Fryman, has put it, a bridge appeared to be created between practitioner and patient.

But from this discovery, explicable in mechanical terms, it was a short step to a further experiment to see what would happen if the hands were placed not on the body, but just above it. And Fryman found they often had the same effect; the muscles and ligaments relaxed. Even if Carpenter's hypersensitivity theory could have been resurrected to account for this phenomenon, it would have brought little comfort to manipulators of the old mechanical school confronted with this evidence.

The belief that osteopathy and chiropractic are specific therapies, which can be taught much as surgery is taught, is consequently becoming untenable. Of course most manipulators continue to practise what they were taught, and to regard the recent developments with some distrust. But the fact that a practitioner has 'DO' or 'DC' after his name now means little more than he originally trained in one school or the other, providing no reliable indication of what he practises. And this is becoming increasingly true of practitioners of all kinds of natural therapies.

Cross-fertilisation is also likely to continue because the marriage between yoga and auto-suggestion is throwing up fresh evidence of the reality of what used to be thought of (or scoffed at) as supernatural phenomena. Another of the experiments undertaken by Elmer Green at the Menninger Foundation has been with Jack Schwartz, who demonstrates that he can drive knitting needles through his biceps without feeling pain or losing blood. This has been a common enough form of exhibitionism in the East, with such variations as the bed of nails or fire walking; but Green decided to try it out in laboratory conditions. As a check, he asked Schwartz to pull a needle out and let the blood flow, which it did; but

Schwartz had only to say 'now it stops' and the flow ceased. Following the tests, the holes left in the skin soon closed up. 'All traces of one puncture had disappeared in twenty-four hours.'

Experiments conducted by Norman Shealy in Wisconsin have had even more spectacular results. When he qualified as a neurosurgeon Shealy became interested in the subject of pain, and invented electrical gadgets to help control it, some of which are still in use. But he was quick to realise the significance of biofeedback and autogenic training for his work with patients, and he began to experiment with a young American psychic, William Neal, who claimed to be able to render himself immune not merely from pain, but also from some of the ordinary consequences of painful experiences such as being burned or beaten. Robert Eagle has described how he watched Neal sticking needles into himself without bleeding; cutting bits of skin off, still without losing blood; holding his hand in a flame; jumping up and down on broken glass in his bare feet; and smashing one pound cans of food down on his fingers hard enough for the cans to buckle. Yet within three hours the skin, where he had cut it or where it had been broken, had healed; and there was no sign of damage to his hands.

Reports of this nature would be harder to credit were it not for the fact that they echo accounts of historical episodes, such as the events at St Médard; and also of shamanist practices. An unexplained, and in everyday terms inexplicable, element remains not just in the healing process, but in the body's capacity to resist injury, which lies outside psychology's normal range.

Conversely, as Emilio Servadio, Professor of Psychology in Genoa University, urged in a paper on the subject in 1963, research into healing will be of no practical use 'unless it is accompanied by a close study of the psychological situation and types of the patients on whom these experiments are carried out', and also of the healer-patient relationships formed. Servadio cited the example of trials of a healer which had been conducted at the Freiburg University over a fourteen-month period in which for the first time psychological types and attitudes had been considered; a preliminary step which he considered very much more important than the actual results of the experiment (they showed that one in ten of patients had shown some objective improvement) because it recognised that for healing to be understood, it will be necessary to find out how psychological and psychic forces interact.

This has since been accepted by the humanistic psychologists, and by Charles Tart, Professor of Psychology at the University of California, in his *Transpersonal Psychologies*. Tart first realised how limited, and even irrelevant, the mechanistic approach can be while he was doing research into altered states of consciousness. A Gallup poll revealed that half the college students in the United States had tried marihuana, and a large proportion used it fairly regularly, in spite of the fact that they risked long prison terms and ruined careers. Why? All that orthodox scientific research had to reveal about marihuana was that it brought about 'a slight increase in heart rate, reddening of the eyes, some difficulty with memory, and small decrements in performance on complex psychomotor tests'; hardly worth risking jail for! But conventional psychiatrists had tended to take the same 'scientific' line, not trusting themselves to admit the reality of any mental or emotional process which cannot be quantified. The transpersonal psychologies now break away from this limitation, emphasising the need to take into consideration all forms of experience whether they be called spiritual, or psychic, or simply left undefined – when searching for ways to promote health and prevent or treat disease.

HOLISM

So vitalism is back: the currently fashionable term for it being holism (some prefer 'wholism'; more self-explanatory, but uglier). Holism, though, is often used in a very limited sense. Presenting acupuncture, chiropractic, herbalism, homeopathy, naturopathy, osteopathy, radionics and healing as worthy of recognition by the British National Health Service, the Healing Research Trust has claimed that they are all 'based on a philosophy of holism'; but so far as most practitioners are concerned all that this means is that they try to treat the patient, rather than simply the patient's symptoms. It rarely impels a chiropractor or acupuncturist to study psychology, let alone healing or radiesthesia. The organisations representing manipulators, in fact, often make little attempt to disguise their impatience with such dabblers in the occult who, they feel, jeopardise the chances of the more scientific therapies obtaining State recognition.

But there is no compelling reason why only organisations should be regarded as acceptable. In the memorandum of evidence to the Royal Commission on the National Health Service, the Healing Research Trust has suggested that Parliament should pass a 'Paramedical Licensing Act', which would simply make provision for the licensing of any 'adequately qualified' individual practitioner; an extension of Shaw's 'Lambeth Degree' idea, though the memorandum does not go into the subject of how the licenses would be awarded. But it goes on to recommend that licensed paramedical practitioners should be remunerated by the Health Service on a 'per item of service' basis. Nothing would be better calculated to bring paramedical practice into disrepute, if healers and radiesthetists were to be at liberty to charge for their services while GPs in the Health Service were not permitted to do so.

'The 'Health for the New Age' Trust's memorandum to the Royal Commission has urged another course: the setting up of Health Centres at which it will be possible to obtain alternative forms of treatment. There is a precedent for this in the San Francisco 'Center for the Study of Health Maintenance Practices', a project which arose out of a students' report, *Autopsy on the American Medical Association*, published in 1970. Aided by a grant from the International Chiropractic Association of California, a group of dedicated San Francisco citizens gave up their spare time to setting up the Center at Berkeley, where it provided the community in general, and University students in particular, with the opportunity to receive a variety of treatments, and attend a variety of courses in preventive medicine: nature cure, chiropractic, massage, t'ai chi, yoga. The Center was immediately successful; too successful, as things turned out, because the founders realised they had taken on more of a job than, as part-timers earning their living elsewhere, they could handle. An attempt was made to convert it into a co-operative; but the practitioners, skilled though they might be in their own therapies, found it impossible to cope with the problems of management.

Projects along these lines, though, probably offer the easiest way in which traditional medicine can be made available to people who want it. Premises do not need to be elaborate: any rambling old house can be adapted for the purpose, with paramedical practitioners renting consulting rooms in it in the same way as specialists do in houses in Harley Street. The 'Health for the New Age' memorandum to the Royal Commission makes the point that such establishments ought not to concentrate simply on providing treatment, but should follow the example of the Peckham Experiment in London between the wars, a Health Centre where the emphasis really was on health, being designed so that families could come for a swim or exercise in a gymnasium, with playrooms for children and parents' gossip-and-tea-rooms, so that the doctors could meet their patients and advise them while they were well, rather than waiting for them to be ill.

The advantage of projects along the lines of the Berkeley Center is that they can begin in a small way, and expand according to the public's need for, and appreciation of, their services. But much will depend on the willingness of the medical profession to forget its former passion for exclusivity, and to recognise the advantages of accepting the practitioners of traditional medicine as potential allies, rather than as rivals. It is not inconceivable that the next stage will be the development of informal local alliances between doctors and acupuncturists, osteopaths, healers and others, so that when backers can be found to set up health centres on the Berkeley or Peckham principle they will be able to offer whatever treatment, orthodox or unorthodox, is required – and, better, instruction in how to avoid the need for treatment.

Postscript

In their *Beyond Biofeedback*, Elmer and Alyce Green recall how they came to be involved in research into the power of the mind to heal the body; and their story can be regarded as a parable for our time.

As a boy, Elmer Green occasionally had dreams which turned out to foreshadow the future; and while at school he came under the influence of a teacher who had studied Sufism and who advocated meditation as a way of training the mind to bring the body under better control. Working as a physicist during the war and in the post-war period, Green had little chance to satisfy the curiosity these experiences had aroused; but eventually he and Alyce, whom he had married, decided to make the break, and to qualify as psychologists. During their courses they came across Schultz and Luthe's *Autogenic Training*, which gave them a line of research which they could pursue – Elmer's background as a physicist enabling him to devise and use the required technological aids; and it was this useful dual qualification which put him in line for a post at the Menninger Foundation in Kansas.

When Elmer arrived for an interview, his first sight of the Foundation 'broke' a well-remembered dream which he had had many years before. The campus was as he had seen it in the dream: a tree-covered hill, buildings, a clock-tower; and the Director turned out to be Gardner Murphy, one of the very few eminent psychologists of recent years to have identified himself with psychical research. Murphy encouraged the Greens to pursue their investigations into biofeedback and autogenic training; and with the help of rigorously scientific tests they were able to confirm that a yogi really could exercise the control over his autonomic nervous system, as legend had maintained. In the process, too, they also learned that Schultz (and Coué) had been right: it is the imagination, not the will, which has to be brought into action to control pulse rate, or blood pressure, or brain rhythms.

The Greens cite many examples of the way in which autogenic training, if necessary coupled with biofeedback, has enabled people to bring down their blood pressure, to relieve or remove their migraine attacks, to control their asthma, and so on. As similar results have been obtained by other researchers in so many different parts of the world, notably in the Centre for Autogenic Training in London, it is difficult to underestimate their importance. If they are accepted, the inescapable implication is that much of what is taught and practised in the medical profession is either unnecessary, in that patients could learn to obtain the same and better results themselves, or positively harmful, in that it inhibits natural healing forces.

This is what has given the practitioners of natural medicine their chance. Some of them, admittedly, are hardly more aware of the significance of what has been learned about the power of auto-suggestion than the most hide-bound physician; many an osteopath or acupuncturist continues to manipulate spines or insert needles according to the book. But in general there is a much greater willingness to accept not just that treatment needs to be related to the patient rather than to the symptoms, but also that whatever the form of treatment may be, if it succeeds it is, as the Greens emphasise, '*the patient who does it*'; most forms of natural medicine can best be regarded as devices, just as biofeedback is, to release the patients' healing potential.

By contrast, the medical profession is less well placed to exploit the discoveries of the past decade. Old prejudices, admittedly, are dying. Scientific and medical journals have recently contained many reports about, say, bioelectricity and biomagnetism, following long years of neglect of their possibilities, a process which may even culminate in the restoration of Mesmer to respectability. The need to accept acupuncture analgesia, too, has led to greater caution in pronouncements about what is, and what is not, 'scientific'. 'Enlightened physicians are not only finding much of obvious value within heterodoxies,' Colin Tudge has observed in the *New Scientist* recently, 'but also feel there may be much more to discover.

The structure of the medical profession, though, militates against incorporation of heterodoxies even when they win acceptance, unless they can be fitted into one of the prevailing specialist empires. Hypnotherapy, manipulation and acupuncture have to be learned, where they are learned at all, after qualification. And the whole bias of medical education, compartmentalised as it is into narrow specialist disciplines concentrating on the treatment of specific sets of symptoms, remains unsuited to the introduction of holistic principles and methods.

What seems most likely to happen is that the medical profession will continue much as before, though with a greater readiness to allow (and even encourage) patients to try alternative methods. This will necessitate, at some stage, legislation to bring the practitioners of natural medicine into State Healh Services, or at least into some form of association with them; perhaps by making more flexible the regulations which already control medical auxiliaries – nurses, psychotherapists, physiotherapists and the rest. Many of them would welcome release from the domination of the medical profession, leaving them with more responsibility for their own decisions, and more scope to use their own initiative.

Here, the work of Dolores Krieger, Professor of Nursing at the University of New York, could provide a precedent. In a careful research project, Krieger was able to show that the laying on of hands by selected nurses did not merely make patients feel better : it significantly altered the value of their hemoglobin (the pigment of the red blood cells which feeds oxygen to the tissues), as if their blood had been given a boost. Nurses whom she has trained have since been applying that traditional technique as part of their work. There would be difficulties in the way of nurses applying it in Britain (though doubtless many of them do, unwittingly); but if they should acquire greater independence under some new charter, the way would be open for them to take a more positive role, perhaps also forming a link between the medical profession and the newcomers.

Reports of recent tests, not yet published, suggest that Matthew Manning can influence enzyme activity in test tubes, and even change the metabolism of cancer cells, by the laboratory equivalent of the laying on of hands: a reminder of the existence of unexplained healing forces over and above those released by auto-suggestion. But here again, orthodox medical scientists, though they have sometimes undertaken to devise and monitor tests, have often been unwilling to accept the results, when favourable. It has been difficult for researchers to find a scientific journal willing to publish their papers (in Manning's case, the researchers themselves have sometimes backed down, uneasy about the prospect of being branded as eccentrics or dupes).

What is needed, then, is a new recruiting system for natural medicine – perhaps for medicine in general – enabling prospective practitioners to qualify on the strength of their talent and their character rather than through the stock academic channels. Not that these should be dispensed with: one sensible idea which has been floated is that a training course should be introduced which anybody who wishes to take up any form of therapy can take, embracing such subjects as biology, psychology and physiology, but including spells of practical study in first aid, social work, hospital posts and so on. Such a course could be regarded not as a hurdle to be surmounted in order to obtain qualification, but as an invaluable introduction to the problems which everybody in this field – acupuncturist or anesthetist, nurse or neurosurgeon – will face.

Acknowledgements: Sources

I am not going to attempt to list all the people who have helped, over the past twenty years, in the course of my researches into unconventional aspects of medicine: many of them correspondents whom I have never met but who have written to recommend some book, pamphlet or article which I could otherwise have missed. My thanks to them all; and to Bernard Levin and Kit Pedler, who undertook to read the proofs.

My greatest debt, however, is to Ruth West, without whose guidance through the maze of natural medicine (as it has become, in the last decade) I should frequently have been baffled. Her knowledge of recent developments in this field is unrivalled; and she has provided the list of organisations which follows the bibliography. She has asked me to point out that if the recent past is any indication it will not be long before some of them will have altered their names or their addresses, some will have split into two or more groups, and some will have merged with others. Where confusion arises as a result, most of the 'umbrella organisations' which she lists can give advice and information.

Bibliography

A recent list of books in print dealing with natural medicine runs to around one thousand five-hundred titles, and more are appearing every month. I have included only those works which are mentioned in the text, or which I have found most useful as general introductions to the aspect with which they are dealing; and many of them provide bibliographies of more specialized books and articles.

The date and place of publication refer to the copy I have consulted, not necessarily to the first edition.

HISTORICAL AND ANTHROPOLOGICAL

Adams, F. (tr.) *Hippocrates*, London 1939
Bramwell, J. M. *Hypnotism*, London 1903
Breuer, J. and Freud, S. *Studies on Hysteria*, London 1956
Coué, Emile *Self-Mastery Through Conscious Suggestion*, London 1922
Eddy, Mary Baker *Science and Healing*, Boston 1902
Eliade, Mircea *Shamanism*, Princeton 1970
Evans-Pritchard, E. E. *Witchcraft, Oracles and Magic among the Azande*, Oxford 1937
Foucault, Michael *The Birth of the Clinic*, New York 1975
Hahnemann, Samuel *Organon of the Rational Art of Healing*, London 1913
Hunter, Richard and Macalpine, Ida *Three Hundred Years of Psychiatry (1535-1860)*, Oxford 1963
Gelfand, Michael *Witch Doctor*, London 1964
Greatrakes, Valentine *Letter to Robert Boyle*, London 1666
Groddeck, Georg *The Unknown Self*, London 1937
Janet, Pierre *Psychological Healing*, London 1925
Lang, Andrew *The Making of Religion*, London 1898
Maclean, Una *Magical Medicine*, London 1971

Bibliography

Millingen, J. G. *Curiosities of Medical Experience*, London 1839

Morley, Mary and Wallis Roys (eds.) *Culture and Caring: Anthropological Perspectives on Traditional Medical Beliefs and Practices*, London 1978

Paget, James *Selected Essays*, London 1902

Peel, Robert *Christian Science*, New York 1958

Rivers, W. H. R. *Medicine, Magic and Religion*, London 1924

Sargant, William *The Mind Possessed*, London 1973

Sigerist, Henry *A History of Medicine*, Oxford 1951

Trilles, H. *Fleurs Noirs et Ames Blanches*, Lille 1914

Tylor, E. B. *Primitive Culture*, London 1871

Tuke, Daniel Hack *Illustrations of the Influence of the Mind upon the Body*, London 1871

Wesley, John *Primitive Physick*, Bristol 1768

Zweig, Stephan *Mental Healers*, New York 1952

CONTEMPORARY

Annett, S. *Ways of Being: A Guide to Spiritual Groups and Growth Centres in Britain*, London 1976

Brelet, Claudine *Guérir Autrement*, Paris 1978

Bricklin, Mark *The Practical Encyclopedia of Natural Healing*, Emmaus (Penn.) 1976

Carlson, Rick (ed.) *The Frontiers of Science and Medicine*, London 1975

Coxhead, Nona *Mindpower*, London 1976

Dixon, Bernard *Beyond the Magic Bullet*, London 1978

Dubos, René *Mirage of Health*, London 1960

Dunbar, Flanders *Mind and Body*, New York 1947

Eagle, Robert *Alternative Medicine*, London 1979

Forbes, Alec *Try Being Healthy*, Plymouth 1976

Graupner, Heinz *Adventures in Healing*, London 1962

Guirdham, Arthur *A Theory of Disease*, London 1957

Hill, Ann *Visual Encyclopedia of Unconventional Medicine*, New York 1979

Holzer, Hans *Beyond Medicine*, New York 1973

Illich, Ivan *Medical Nemesis*, London 1975

Langdon-Davis, John   *Man: The Known and Unknown*, London 1960
La Patra, Jack   *Healing: The Coming Revolution in Holistic Medicine*, New York 1978
Lasagna, Louis   *The Doctors' Dilemmas*, New York 1962
Murray, Geoffrey   *Frontiers of Healing*, London 1958
Palaiseul, Jean   *Au Déla De La Médecine: Tous Les Moyens De Vous Guérir Interdits Aux Medécins*, Paris 1958
Pauwels, Louis (ed.)   *Les Médecines Différentes*, Paris 1970
Popenoe, Cris   *Wellness*, Washington 1977
Selye, Hans   *The Stress of Life*, New York 1956
Simeons, A. T. W.   *Man's Presumptuous Brain*, London 1960
Smith, Adam   *Powers of Mind*, New York 1975
Thomson, William A. R.   *The Searching Mind in Medicine*, London 1960
Watson, Lyall   *Lifetide*, London 1979
Weatherhead, Leslie   *Psychology, Religion and Healing*, London 1951
Wilson, Colin   *Mysteries*, London 1978

ACUPUNCTURE

Academy of Traditional Chinese Medicine   *An Outline of Chinese Acupuncture*, Peking 1975
Austin, Mary   *Textbook of Acupuncture Therapy*, London 1972
Mann, Felix   *Acupuncture*, London 1962
Melzack, Ronald   *The Puzzle of Pain*, London 1973
Talof, Stephan   *The Chinese Art of Healing*, New York 1972
Veith, Ilza   *The Yellow Emperor's Classic of Internal Medicine*, London 1972
Wu Wei-Ping   *Chinese Acupuncture*, Wellingborough (Northants) 1974

HEALING: SPIRITUAL, PSYCHIC, ESOTERIC

Academy of Science and Medicine   *The Varieties of Healing Experience*, Los Angeles 1972
Archbishops' Commission Report   *The Church's Ministry of Healing*, London 1958

Bibliography

Bailey, Alice A. *Esoteric Healing*, New York and London 1953

Barbanell, Maurice *I Hear a Voice: A Biography of Ted Fricker*, London 1962

Edwards, Harry *Spirit Healing*, London 1960

Fox, Alfred Purcell *The Church's Ministry of Healing*, London 1959

Fuller, J. G. *Arigo*, New York 1974

Greene, Liz *Relating*, New York 1977

Guirdham, Arthur *The Nature of Healing*, London 1964

Krippner, Stanley and Villoldo, Alberto *The Realms of Healing*, Millbrae (Cal.) 1976

LeShan, Lawrence *The Medium, the Mystic and the Physicist*, New York 1974

MacNutt, Francis *The Power to Heal*, Indiana 1977

Meek, George W. *Healers and the Healing Process*, Illinois 1977

Millard, Joseph *Edgar Cayce*, London 1961

Netherton, Maurice and Shiffrin, Nancy *Past Lives Therapy*, New York 1978

Playfair, Guy *The Flying Cow*, London 1975

Rose, Louis *Faith Healing*, London 1968

Servadio, Emilio *Unconscious and Paranormal Factors in Healing and Recovery*, London 1963

Shealy, Norman *Occult Medicine Can Save Your Life*, New York 1975

Sherman, Harold *Wonder Healers of the Philippines*, London 1967 (New York 1960)

Theosophical Research Centre Medical Group *The Mystery of Healing*, London 1958

Thompson, C. J. S. *Magic and Healing*, London 1946

Worral, A. A. and Worral, Olga *The Gift of Healing*, New York 1965

HERBALISM

Chancellor, P. M. *Handbook of the Bach Flower Remedies*, London 1971

Conway, J. *The Magic of Herbs*, London 1973

Culpeper, Nicholas *English Physician and Complete Herbal* (ed. Mrs C. F. Leyel), London 1961

Grieve, M. *A Modern Herbal*, London 1976

Hyatt, Richard *Chinese Herbal Medicine*, London 1978

Leyel, Hilda (Mrs C. F.) *Green Medicine*, London 1952

Thomson, William A. R. *Herbs that Heal*, London 1976

Weeks, Nora *The Medical Discoveries of Edward Bach*, London 1940

HOMEOPATHY

Blackie, Margery *The Patient, not the Cure*, London 1976

Bott, V. *Anthroposophical Medicine*, London 1978

Coulter, Harris *Homeopathic Medicine*, London 1975

Gibson, D. M. *First Aid Homeopathy*, London 1975

Mitchell, G. Ruthven *Homeopathy*, London 1975

Speight, Phyllis *Homeopathy: A Practical Guide to Natural Medicine*, London 1979

MANIPULATIVE THERAPIES: OSTEOPATHY, CHIROPRACTIC, ETC

Alexander, F. Matthias *The Universal Constant in Living*, New York 1941

Barker, Herbert *Leaves from My Life*, London 1927

Barlow, Wilfred *The Alexander Principle*, London 1973

Dummer, Thomas G. *Out on the Fringe*, London 1963

Korr, Irvin *The Physiological Basis of Osteopathic Medicine*, New York 1970

Lowen, Alexander *The Betrayal of the Body*, New York 1967

Rolf, Ida *'Structural Integration' Systematics, Vol. 1* 1963

Schafer, R. C. *Chiropractic Health Care*, Des Moynes (Iowa) 1976

Still, Andrew Taylor *Autobiography*, Kirksville (Mo.) 1908

Stoddard, Alan *Manual of Osteopathic Practice*, London 1969

Weiant, C. W. and Goldschmidt, S. *Medicine and Chiropractic*, New York 1959

NATURE CURE : NATUROPATHY

Davis, Adelle *Let's Get Well*, New York 1965

Jarvis, D. C. *Folk Medicine*, New York 1958

Lederman, E. K. *Good Health Through Natural Therapy*, London 1976

Moyle, Alan *About Nature Cure*, London 1965

Turner, E. S. *Taking the Cure*, London 1967

Warmbrand, Max *The Encyclopedia of Health and Nutrition*, New York 1962

PSYCHOTHERAPEUTIC TECHNIQUES : AUTO-SUGGESTION, AUTOGENIC TRAINING, HYPNOSIS, BIOFEEDBACK, ETC

Assagioli, Roberto *Psychosynthesis*, New York 1965

Benson, Herbert *The Relaxation Response*, London 1976

Berne, Eric *Games People Play*, London 1968

Black, S. *Mind and Body*, London 1969

Blythe, Peter *Self-Hypnotism*, London 1976

Brown, Barbara B. *Stress and the Art of Biofeedback*, New York 1978

Bry, Adelaide *Est*, New York 1976

Cade, C. Maxwell and Coxhead, Nona *The Awakened Mind*, New York 1979

Ehrenwald, Jan *Telepathy and Medical Psychology*, London 1948

Green, Elmer and Green, Alyce *Beyond Biofeedback*, New York 1977

Hargrove, Robert *Est: Making Life Work*, New York 1976

Hubbard, L. Ron *Dianetics*, London 1960

Hutchinson, Ronald *Yoga*, London 1974

Jaffe, Denis T. *In Search of a Therapy*, New York 1975

Janov, Arthur *The Primal Revolution*, London 1975

Kaslof, Leslie J. *Wholistic Dimensions in Healing*, New York 1978

Laing, Ronald D. *The Divided Self*, London 1960

Maharishi Mahesh Yoga *The Science of Being*, London 1966

Maslow, A. H. *The Farther Reaches of Human Nature*, London 1976

Ornstein, Robert E. *The Nature of Human Consciousness*, San Francisco 1973

Owen, A. R. G. *Hysteria, Hypnosis and Healing*, London 1971

Pelletier, Kenneth R. *Mind as Healer, Mind as Slayer*, New York 1977

Perls, Fritz *Gestalt Therapy*, New York 1951

Rogers, Carl *On Becoming a Person*, London 1962

Schultz, J. H. and Luthe, W. *Autogenic Training*, New York 1959

Shattlock, E. H. *Mind Your Body*, London 1979

Silva, Jose *The Silva Mind Control Method*, London 1978

Tart, Charles *Transpersonal Psychologies*, New York 1975

Wolff, Harold *Stress and Disease*, Springfield (Ill.) 1968

RADIONICS, RADIESTHESIA

Ash, Michael *Health, Radiation and Healing*, London 1962

Day, L. and De La Warr, G. *New Worlds Beyond the Atom*, London 1956

Drown, Ruth *The Science and Philosophy of the Drown Radio Therapy*, Los Angeles 1938

Mermet, Abbé *Principles and Practice of Radiesthesia*, London 1935

Reyner, J. H. *Psionic Medicine*, London 1974

Tansley, David *Radionics*, Devon 1972

Watson T. T. B. *Radiesthesia and some Associated Phenomena*, London 1954

Westlake, Aubrey *The Pattern of Health*, London 1961

Wilcox, John *Radionic Theory and Practice*, London 1960

Names and Addresses of Organisations Involved in the Practice of Natural Medicine

CONTENTS

The date in brackets is when each organisation was founded in the UK. Organisations would appreciate an s.a.e. from anyone requesting further information

N.B.: All figures given are approximate; membership numbers are for the UK only unless otherwise stated

† Indicates medical organisation

1. UMBRELLA ORGANISATIONS AND THE MAIN NETWORKS

Foundations and trusts

Action for Natural Therapies (1980)
c/o 7 Regency Terrace, London SW7 3QW. Tel. 01-370 3651.
Aim: 'to increase the public's knowledge of natural therapies and widen their availability; to maintain the freedom to practise natural therapies that at present exists in the UK; to help bridge the gap between natural therapies and technical medicine.'

Healing Research Trust (1974)
An extension of the Keys Trust (1967) c/o Heseltine Moss and Co., 3/4 Trump Street, London EC2V 8DH.
Aim: 'to promote alternative medicine, encourage systematic research in healing techniques and provide grants for education.'

Health for the New Age (1972)
1a Addison Crescent, London W14 8JP. Tel. 01-603 7751.
Aim: 'to encourage the growth of holistic health care, the exchange of information between groups and individuals concerned with health, the promotion of research.' Newsletter.

National Association for Health (1960)
Greenways, Hillview Road, Claygate, Surrey KT10 0TU. Tel. 78 64633.
Aim: 'to be an advisory and independent "watchdog" on matters affecting the public health, especially regarding medicines and foods.'

Threshold Foundation (1978)
7 Regency Terrace, London SW7 3QW. Tel. 01-370 3651.
Aim: 'to promote a holistic approach to the understanding of the universe through research, educational and cultural activities.' Administers an annual award of $50,000.

World Federation of Life Sciences (1974)
  25 Chapel Street, St Kilda, Victoria 3182, Australia.
  Aim: to co-ordinate 'and promote the work of non-orthodox
  medical and health disciplines, world-wide.'

Wrekin Trust (1971)
  Dove House, Little Birch, Hereford HR 2 8BB. Tel. 09814
  224.
  Residential weekend seminars, workshops and conferences
  around the country on 'biofeedback and self-awareness',
  transpersonal psychology, dowsing and healing, astrology
  and psychology of relationships, western mystery traditions,
  etc. Annual conference on 'health and healing'. Mailing list,
  newsletter.

Practitioner and Client Organisations

Association for Humanistic Psychology (1972)
  62 Southwark Bridge Road, London SE1 0AU. Tel. 01-928
  8254.
  Open to anyone interested in the human potential movement. Conferences, seminars, workshops. Information on
  practitioners in UK. Journal. Members: 450 including
  overseas.

British Committee for Natural Therapeutics (1968)
  c/o 39 Harley Street, London W1. Tel. 01-580 4706.
  Aim 'to represent all the organisations in natural medicine
  of accepted professional standing.' Member organisations: 5
  (British members of IFPNT).

International Federation of Practitioners of Natural
Therapeutics (1965)
  c/o 39 Harley Street, London W1. Tel. 01-580 4706.
  In a 'working relationship' with the World Health Organisation. Represents the interests of 40 organisations in 14
  member countries.

The Patients Association (1963)
 11 Dartmouth Street, London SW1H 9BN. Tel. 01-222
 4992.
 Aim: 'to represent and further the interest of patients.'
 Advice service; campaigns for improvements in the NHS.
 Newsletter, bulletin, information leaflets. Members: 800.

Research Society for Natural Therapeutics (1959)
 8 Stokewood Road, Bournemouth BH3 7NA. Tel. 0202
 25997.
 Postgraduate courses, seminars in cranial osteopathy, irid-
 ology, etc.; research by individual members. Journal.
 Members: 80 practitioners, 60 associates.

Networks

Positive Health Network (1978)
 29 Meads Street, Eastbourne, Sussex BN20 7RH. Tel. 0323
 26022.
 'An alliance of many groups concerned with community and
 personal responsibility for health and with complementary
 therapies.' Members: 35.

Scientific and Medical Network (1973)
 Lake House, Ockley, Nr Dorking, Surrey RH5 5NS. Tel.
 0306 711268.
 'Share the conviction that the contemporary framework of
 thought in science and medicine should be widened to
 include certain ideas that go beyond what today is considered orthodox.' Newsletters, research, seminars, annual
 May lectures. Members: 200 in academic and scientific
 posts (by invitation only).

2. CENTRES FOR TREATMENT AND EDUCATION

Anthroposophical Society in Great Britain (1920s)
Rudolf Steiner House, 35 Park Road, London NW1 6XT.
Tel. 01-723 4400.
Based on the teachings of Rudolf Steiner, offers the following facilities: School of Eurythmy (4-year diploma course); School of Speech Formation (3–4-year diploma course); courses in drama, painting. Curative education – 26 homes and schools for physically and mentally handicapped, 4 for maladjusted, 6 village communities for handicapped adults; Anthroposophical Medicine Association. Full-time courses in anthroposophy at Emerson College (1962), Forest Row, Sussex RH18 5JX. Tel. 034282 2238. Students: 100 foundation course; 35 teacher training; 20 social development. Quarterly and annual journals.

Claregate College (1977)
Great North Road, Little Heath, Potters Bar EN6 1JI.
Tel. 77 42341.
One-day and weekend courses on esoteric healing, science, psychology and astrology. Offers Degree of Bachelor of Metaphysics. Journal.

College of Psychic Studies (1884)
16 Queensbury Place, London SW7 2EB. Tel. 01-589 3292.
Lecture programme, psychological and personal counselling, distant healing, workshops on: transpersonal psychology, altered states of consciousness, 'psychic unfoldment'; courses in: t'ai chi' meditation, on reincarnation, teachings from the spiritual world etc. Training for mediumship; demonstrations of clairvoyance, etc. Library. Journal. Members: 800.

Community Health Foundation (1976), incorporating the East West Centre & Michio Kushi Institute.
188 Old Street, London EC1V 9BP. Tel. 01-251 4076.
Aim: 'to teach practical preventive medicine in the community and to publish results of research arising from educational projects.' Classes and discussion groups on

nutrition, shiatsu, massage, reflexology, hatha yoga, t'ai chi, macrobiotics, oriental diagnosis. The 'Growing Family Centre'. Journal. Members: 500.

The Findhorn Foundation (1962)
The Park, Forres IV36 0TZ. Tel. 055581 311.
An educational and spiritual working community, and New Age centre of education. Resident members and guests: 300.

Friends of the Healing Research Trust (1977)
1 Castle Street, Totnes, Devon.
Aim: to promote and encourage the growth of natural health centres which offer advice and treatment 'by as many different therapies as are available in each neighbourhood'. Centres: 15 (orthodox doctors are co-operating). Newsletter. Members: 1300.

Health Farms/Centres
For an up-to-date list see the *International Vegetarian Health Food Handbook* (available from the Vegetarian Society).

The Kent House Centre (1977)
Camden Park, Tunbridge Wells, Kent TN2 5AN. Tel. 0892 36709.
'Training in techniques of contemplative prayer and meditation'; 'facilities for the study of wholeness in relation to medicine and the healing ministry'; 'a place for individual and group retreats'.

Salisbury Centre (1973)
2 Salisbury Road, Edinburgh EH16 5AB. Tel. 031-667 5438.
An open community. Programme includes analysis and therapy groups, t'ai chi, hatha yoga, astrology, meditation, pottery, weaving. Visitors welcome.

The above 2 centres are also members of a network of 'open centres'. Aim: 'to be open to the truth through silence, meditation and healing'. For information about other such groups contact: Avils Farm, Lower Stanton, Chippenham, Wiltshire. Tel. 0249 720202. Newsletter.

Leamington Spa Health Foundation (1977)

c/o 21 Mason Road, Lillington, Leamington Spa, Warwickshire. Tel. 0926 44279.

Aim: 'to provide opportunities for local people to learn about self-help in positive health.' Evening classes (at low prices) in massage, relaxation, women's health, organic gardening, t'ai chi, etc.

Manjushri Institute (1976)

Conishead Priory, Ulverston, Cumbria LA12 9QQ. Tel. 0229 54019.

Short courses, group retreats, weekend seminars – run by 'fully qualified Tibetan masters' and western students of Buddhism – on Tibetan medicine, Buddhism and western psychology, health and meditation, tantric yoga, etc. London Centre.

For other Buddhist centres offering courses in yoga, meditation, psychology, apply to: The Buddhist Society, 58 Eccleston Square, London SW1V 1PH. Tel. 01-828 1313.

The Nature Cure Clinic (1928)

15 Oldbury Place, London W1M 3AL. Tel. 01-935 2787. Clinic 'for patients with limited means'. Staff includes doctors, naturopaths, osteopaths and homeopaths.

The Portland Centre (1978)

16 Preston Street, Brighton, Sussex. Tel. 0273 27464.

Bookshop. Facilities for healing, relaxation therapy, natural therapies (acupuncture, auricular therapy, reflexology, chiropractic). Seminars.

Ramana Health Centre (1975)

Ludshott Manor Hospital, Bramshott, Liphook, Hampshire GU30 7RD. Tel. 0428 722993.

Aim: to combine the best of conventional medicine with natural therapies: homeopathy, nature cure, acupuncture, osteopathy, chiropractic, radionics, spiritual healing, etc. 16 beds. Medical supervision. Members: 200.

Saros (1979)

Hardwick Hall, Hardwick Square, South Buxton, Derbyshire.

Foundation for 'the perpetuation of knowledge'. Courses in tarot, meditation, Buddhism, kabbalah, calligraphy, astrology, etc. Activities also in Cambridge (0223 65864), London (01-431 1407), Manchester (061-861 9523), Oxford (0865 57876).

Totnes Natural Health Centre (1978)

1 Castle Street, Totnes, Devon. Tel. 0803 864 587.

Aim: education and information on natural medicine. Group or individual relaxation and counselling facilities.

The Wellbeing Centre (1979)

Old School House, Churchtown, 1 Hogan, Redruth, Cornwall. Tel. 0209 842 999.

Newly established trust concerned with 'self-healing'.

Wessex Healthy Living Foundation (1977)

72 Belle Vue Road, Southbourne, Bournemouth BH6 3DX. Tel. 0202 422087.

Natural therapeutics clinic, at present offers osteopathy, aromatherapy, homeopathy, chiropractic, reflexology, acupuncture, massage, naturopathy at reduced fees. Lectures and demonstrations on natural therapies, vegetarian cooking, yoga, meditation, etc. Members: 330.

Westbank Healing and Teaching Centre (1959)

Strathmiglo, Fife KY14 7QP. Tel. 03376 233.

'On-going weekly facilities for training and experience in healing', hatha yoga, meditation, zone therapy, etc. Some accommodation. Monthly courses and healing sessions in London.

Appendix

3. NATURAL THERAPIES

Herbal Medicine

British Herbal Medicine Association (1971)
Lane House, Cowling, Nr Keighley, West Yorkshire BD22 0LX. Tel. 0535 34487.
Aim: to protect the interests of users, practitioners, manufacturers of herbal medicine. Publishes the British Herbal Pharmacopoeia. Members: 141 practitioners and others, 23 companies.

The Faculty of Herbal Medicine (1939)
'Merlynn', 93 East Avenue, Bournemouth BA3 7BK. Tel. 0202 764146.
Correspondence course and practical training. Also offers correspondence courses in osteopathy, physiotherapy, psychology, naturopathy, homeopathy. Members: 500 (British Herbalists Union).

The Herb Society (1927) (originally the Society of Herbalists)
34 Boscobel Place, London, SW1. Tel. 01-235 1023.
Aim: 'to promote, improve and increase the knowledge and use of herbs.' Lectures, outings, library, journal. Members: 1500.

National Institute of Medical Herbalists (1864)
65 Frant Road, Tunbridge Wells, Kent TN2 5LH. Tel. 0892 27439.
A professional body for graduates of the Tutorial School of Herbal Medicine. Members: 100 (MNIMH).

Tutorial School of Herbal Medicine
148 Forrest Road, Tunbridge Wells, Kent. Tel. 0892 30400.
Courses: 4-year full-time home study, including 16 weekend seminars, 4-year full-time attendance. Students: 250.

A course of lectures on 'the art of using herbs safely in daily life' is run according to demand at 14 Ferncroft Avenue, London NW3. Tel. 01-435 9581.

Herbal Remedies

The Herb Society publishes a list of herb growers and suppliers. For a list of over 600 health food stores in the UK, most of which supply herbal remedies, see the *International Vegetarian Health Food Handbook.*

Flower Healing

The Dr Edward Bach Centre (1936)
Mount Vernon, Sotwell, Wallingford, Oxon OX10 0PZ. Tel. 0491 39489.
Send for remedies, books, advice on treatment. For introductory courses on diagnosing, prescribing and healing with the remedies: Melodie Reinhart c/o above address.

Exultation of Flowers (1956)
Seaweed Croft, Geddes, Nairn, Scotland. Tel. 06677 276.
Recommended for first aid and any type of illness.

Vita Florum (1956)
Cats Castle, Lydeard St Lawrence, Taunton, Somerset TA4 3QA. Tel. 09847 329.
A blend of flowers which channels healing. 'Useful in almost every type of illness, mental or physical.'

Aromatherapy

'Works by the action of essential oils on the body and mind.' The oils can be used internally, in massage, and for cosmetic value.

Aromatherapy Training Centre
4 Eltham Road, London SE12. Tel. 01-852 7591.
Courses: 3-day 'intensives' for physiotherapists, nurses, beauty therapists. Keeps list of 150 therapists in UK.

Appendix

Naturopathy

British College of Naturopathy and Osteopathy (1938)
 Frazer House, 6 Netherhall Gardens, London NW3. Tel.
 01-435 8728.
 Courses: 4 years' full-time attendance leading to ND DO.
 Students: 80.

British Naturopathic and Osteopathic Association (1925)
 Frazer House, 6 Netherhall Gardens, London NW3. Tel.
 01-435 8728.
 Publishes a register. Journal. Members: 200 (MBNOA).

Society for the Promotion of Natural Health
 Frazer House, 6 Netherhall Gardens, London NW3. Tel.
 01-435 8728.
 Lay support body for the College and Association. Journal.
 Members: 500.

Diet, Nutrition

† The McCarrison Society (1966)
 23 Stanley Court, Worcester, Sutton, Surrey. Tel. 0734
 473165.
 Founded to study the relation between nutrition and
 health. Members: 300 (medical and allied professions).

Nutrition Science Research Institute (1974)
 Mulberry Tree Hall, Brookthorpe, Gloucestershire GL4
 0UU. Tel. 0452 813471.
 Radiesthetic analysis of 'deficiencies and excesses of nutrients
 and non-nutrients in daily food from an imbalanced diet'
 which lead to disease. Courses on nutrition science.

East West Centre
 (see under 'Centres': *Community Health Foundation*.)
 Courses in macrobiotic nutrition and medicine.

The Vegan Society (1944)
47 Highlands Road, Leatherhead, Surrey. Tel. 03723 72389.
Meetings (including regional ones), publications, advice, etc.
Journal. Members. over 2000 in 26 countries.

The Vegetarian Society (1847)
53 Marloes Road, London W8 6LA. Tel. 01-937 7739.
Cookery courses, lectures, conferences. 40 branches in the
UK. International Vegetarian Health Food Handbook
(annual). Journal. Members: 7000.

Childbirth

Association for Improvements in Maternity Services (1960)
19 Broomfield Crescent, Leeds LS6 3DD. Tel. 0532 751911.
Aim: 'to inform women about the state of maternity care;
to give support and advice on maternity problems.' Campaign to reduce routine inductions and episiotomies. Newsletter. Members: 500. 10 regional groups.

Association of Radical Midwives (1976)
Harringey Women's Centre, 40 Turnpike Lane, London N8.
Tel. 01-889 3912.
Aim: to promote midwifery skills within the community.
Newsletter. Members: 200.

National Childbirth Trust (1956)
9 Queensborough Terrace, London W2 3TB. Tel. 01-229
9319.
Ante-natal classes, breastfeeding counselling, etc. 100 UK
branches. Members: 5000.

Natural Birth Control (1976)
c/o The Public House Bookshop, 21 Little Preston Street,
Brighton BN1 2HQ. Tel. 0273 28357.
Provides monthly charts (plus instructions) for calculating
fertility cycles.

Appendix

Natural Birth Control Consultancy (1978)
14 Bristol Gardens, London W9. Tel. 01-286 0066.
Calculates natal charts and biological rhythms for fertility periods.

Dance Therapy

London School of Eurythmy
(see under 'Centres': Anthroposophical Society).

The Natural Dance Workshop (1975)
Playspace, Peto Place, London NW1 4DT. Tel. 01-278 6783.
'Independent social arts project' to explore, develop and establish natural dance. Runs courses and workshops.

T'ai Chi Chuan

British T'ai Chi Chuan Association and London T'ai Chi Academy (1967)
7 Upper Wimpole Street, London W1. Tel. 01-935 8444.
Teaches the Yang-style, with emphasis on meditation and health. Beginners' course (10 weeks), advanced, teacher training (3 years), healing (6 years). Centres also in Norwich and Powys. Students: 120.

International T'ai Chi Chuan Association
40 Hillcroft Crescent, Wembley Park, Middlesex. Tel. 01-905 2351.
Aim: control of physical energies and disciplining of the personality. Yang-style group and individual sessions.

School of T'ai Chi Chuan (1973)
49 The Avenue, London NW6. Tel. 01-459 0764.
'Oriented for spiritual unfoldment as well as physical reform.' Branches in Birmingham and Leamington Spa.

Eyesight

Bates Association of Eyesight Training (1954)
49 Queen Anne Street, London W1. Tel. 01-935 9847.
Eye defects helped by teaching the art of seeing as 'relaxed attention'. Teachers: 12.

Iris Diagnosis

Based on the principle that 'each organ of the body is represented by an area of the iris' (colour, texture, pattern of the iris are observed).
Courses at the *Community Health Foundation* (see under 'Centres'). For practitioners of natural medicine, weekend courses are given at 46 Kidbrooke Park Road, London SE3. Tel. 01-856 0644. See also under 'Umbrella Organisations': *Research Society for Natural Therapeutics.*

Music Therapy

British Society for Music Therapy (1958)
48 Lanchester Road, London N6 4TA. Tel. 01-883 1331.
Aim: to promote music therapy in the treatment, education, rehabilitation of those suffering from emotional, physical or mental handicap. Journal. Members: 500.

The Nordoff Robbins Music Therapy Centre (1974).
6 Queensdale Walk, London W11 4QQ.
Courses: 1-year full-time for professional musicians (run jointly with the Roehampton Institute of Higher Education). Students: 10 each course.

Colour Therapy

Hygeia Studios (1971)
Brook House, Avening, Tetbury, Gloucestershire, GL8 8NS. Tel. 045383 2150.
Residential courses on the therapeutic aspects of the colour-light art, geometry research that takes place at the studios.

4. HOMEOPATHY

† The Faculty of Homeopathy (1844) (originally the British Homeopathic Society)
   Hahnemann House, 2 Powis Place, Great Ormond Street, London WC1N 3HR. Tel. 01-837 3091.
   The professional body for homeopathic doctors (UK practising: 122 associates; 96 members; 18 fellows), dentists (70), nurses (13) and pharmacists (21). Keeps a register. Courses per year: full-time (10 students); 3 one-week courses (70–5 students) – held at The School of Homeopathy. Requirement for associateship: 6 one-week courses, plus 6 months' clinical. Journal.

† The Homeopathic Trust for Research and Education (1948)
   Hahnemann House, 2 Powis Place, Great Ormond Street, London WC1 3HR. Tel. 01-837 3091.
   Responsible for the continuation of homeopathic research, education and practice. Primarily a fund-raising body.

† Anthroposophical Medical Association (see under 'Centres')
   'A group of registered medical practitioners who practise anthroposophical medicine.' 'Also an initiative group of young doctors and medical students organising biannual conferences.'

British Homeopathic Association (1909)
   27a Devonshire Street, London W1N 1RJ. Tel. 01-935 2163.
   Primarily for lay people. Books and information – including lists of homeopathic doctors, hospitals, and of chemists supplying homeopathic remedies. Courses on first aid and homeopathy. Journal. Members: 2000.

Hahnemann Society (1958)
   Humane Education Centre, Avenue Lodge, Bounds Green Road, London N22 4EU. Tel. 01-889 1595.
   Aim: to advance the education of the public in the principles underlying homeopathic practice. For lay supporters of homeopathy. Newsletter. Members: 1000.

The College of Homeopathy (1978)
  29 Coleraine Road, Blackheath, London SE3. Tel. 01-858 7338.
  Course: 4-year diploma (part-time). Affiliated to the Society of Homeopaths. Students: 30 (first year).

The Society of Homeopaths (1978)
  59 Norfolk House, Streatham, London SW16. Tel. 01-677 3260.
  Aim: to establish a register for fully qualified practitioners of homeopathy by examination and to encourage the growth of the practice of homeopathy as a 'complete and independent system of natural medicine'. Journal. Members: 100.

† Homeopathic Hospitals, Out-Patients and Regional Clinics in the National Health Service
  NB: Although included under the NHS, for homeopathic treatment it is necessary to ask to be referred to a homeopathic physician – otherwise treatment will be given along orthodox lines.

The Royal London Homeopathic Hospital
  Great Ormond Street, London WC1N 3HR. Tel. 01-837 3091.

Glasgow Homeopathic Hospital
  1000 Great Western Road, Glasgow W2. Tel. 041-339 0382.

Glasgow Homeopathic Hospital for Children
  221 Hamilton Road, Glasgow E2. Tel. 041-778 1185.

Glasgow Homeopathic Out-Patient Department
  5 Lynedoch Crescent, Glasgow C3. Tel. 041-332 4490.

The Liverpool Clinic
  1 Myrtle Street, Liverpool L7 7DE. Tel. 061-709 5475.

Bristol Homeopathic Hospital
  Cotham, Bristol 6. Tel. 0272 33068-9.

Tunbridge Wells Homeopathic Hospital
  Church Road, Tunbridge Wells, Kent. Tel. 0892 26111.

Homeopathic Remedies

  Any person may buy or prescribe any remedy, providing it
  is not on the restricted sales list, or one of the 6 or so
  remedies listed as poisonous if given in potencies under
  6x. All remedies are available on the NHS. For names and
  addresses of about 100 chemists in the UK supplying
  homeopathic remedies, apply to the *British Homeopathic
  Association.*

5. OSTEOPATHY AND CHIROPRACTIC; MANIPULATION AND MASSAGE

Osteopathy

† London College of Osteopathic Medicine (1946)
  8-10 Boston Place, London NW2. Tel. 01-262 1128.
  Courses: 13-month full-time for doctors only leading to
  MLCO. Students: 4.

† British Osteopathic Association (1911)
  8-10 Boston Place, London NW2. Tel. 01-262 1128.
  Runs a clinic. Members: 100.

† Osteopathic Medical Association
  c/o 22 Wimpole Street, London W1. Tel. 01-580 6147.
  Members: 10.

British School of Osteopathy (1917)
  16 Buckingham Gate, London SW1E 6LB. Tel. 01-828 9479.
  Courses: 4-year full-time leading to DO. Students: 90.

General Council and Register of Osteopaths (1936)
16 Buckingham Gate, London SW1E 6LB. Tel. 01-828 0601.
Members: 340 (22 abroad) MROs. Graduates of the
London College of Osteopathy and the British School of
Osteopathy are eligible for membership. Keeps a register.

British Naturopathic and Osteopathic Association and College
(see under 'Natural Therapies: Naturopathy').

Ecole Européenne d'Ostéopathie (1974)
104 Tonbridge Road, Maidstone, Kent. Tel. 0622 671558.
Courses: 4-year full-time, leading to DO. Students: 81.
5-year tutorial course in osteopathy (leading to DO) for
French-speaking physiotherapists and natural medicine practitioners. Students: 250.

Society of Osteopaths (1971)
c/o 12 College Road, Eastbourne, East Sussex BN21 4HZ.
Tel. 0323 638606.
Members: 75 (MSO) graduates of Ecole Européenne
d'Ostéopathie. Postgraduate courses. Journal.

Part-time Courses

Andrew Still College of Osteopathy and Natural Therapeutics
(1977)
94 Banstead Road South, Sutton, Surrey. Tel. 01-642 4161.
Courses: 5-year minimum part-time for mature students
leading to DO. Students: 3; postgraduate courses for
osteopaths and physiotherapists e.g. in cranial osteopathy.

College of Osteopathy and Manipulative Therapy (1948)
21 Manor Road North, Wallington, Surrey SM6 7MS. Tel.
01-647 2452.
Courses: 5-year part-time, leading to DO. Students: 45.
Register of members. Members 64 (MCO).

Cranial Osteopathic Association (1968)
  c/o Hatton House, Church Lane, Cheshunt, Hertfordshire
  EN8 0DW. Tel. 97 32085.
  Courses: postgraduate (12 weekends) Students: 15.
  Seminars. Members: 50 (MCrOA).

British and European Osteopathic Association (1976)
  133 Gatley Road, Gatley, Cheadle, Cheshire. Tel. 061-428
  4980.
  An independent body, accepting members from 6 schools of
  osteopathy. Register of members. All are expected to
  undertake regular postgraduate studies. Members: 100
  (BEOA).

Chiropractic

Anglo-European College of Chiropractic (1965)
  1 Cavendish Road, Bournemouth BH1 1QX. Tel 0202
  24777.
  Courses: 4-year full-time leading to DC. Students: 116.

British Chiropractors' Association (1925)
  5 First Avenue, Chelmsford, Essex CM1 1RX. Tel. 0245
  353078.
  Keeps a register of members. Members: 110 DCs (graduates
  of Anglo-European College of Chiropractic).

Oxfordshire School of Chiropractic (1979)
  8 Dashwood Road, Banbury, Oxfordshire. Tel. 0295 2816.
  Courses: 3-year part-time leading to DC. Students: 8.
  2-year part-time for animal therapy. Students: 4.

The Chiropractic Advancement Association (1965)
  38 The Island, Thames Ditton, Surrey KT7 0SQ. Tel. 01-398
  2098. Lay support association. News bulletin, handbook.
  Members: 2000.

Alexander

Alexander Teaching Associates (1980)
  A.T.A. Centre, 188 Old Street, London EC1V 9BP. Tel.
  01-250 3038.
  Individual tuition: evening and weekend classes.

The Constructive Teaching Centre (1946)
  18 Lansdowne Road, London W11. Tel. 01-727 7222.
  Courses: 3-year full-time. Students: 30.

Macdonald's Training Course for the Alexander Technique
(1956)
  50a Belgrave Road, London SW1. Tel. 01-821 7916.
  Courses: 3-year full-time. Students: 26.

The School of Alexander Studies (1975)
  61a Onslow Gardens, London N10. Tel. 01-883 7659.
  Courses: 3-year full-time. Students: 28.

The Society of Teachers of the Alexander Technique (1955)
  3 Albert Court, Kensington Gore, London SW7. Tel. 01-
  589 3834.
  Keeps a register of those qualifying from the above 3
  schools. Journal. Members: 90 (UK), 50 (abroad).

Manipulation

† International Federation of Manual Medicine (1965)
  28 Wimpole Street, London W1M 7AD. Tel. 01-580 0391.
  14 national associations; membership open to those qualified to practise medicine in their own countries. Congress
  every 3rd year.

†British Association of Manipulative Medicine (1968)
  22 Wimpole Street, London W1. Tel. 01-580 4154.
  Weekend courses, for doctors only: 5 per year, held at
  the Brook Hospital (London).

Massage

Andrew Still College of Osteopathy and Natural Therapeutics
94 Banstead Road South, Sutton, Surrey. Tel. 01-642 4161.
Part-time courses in therapeutic massage and soft tissue
manipulation (12 sessions); applied kinesiology (10 weekends). Students: 5.

Churchill Centre (1973)
22 Montagu Street, London W1H 1TB. Tel. 01-402 9475.
Courses: 3 weekends or 12 evenings, practical; 4 theory
sessions for examination leading to diploma in massage.
Students: 8–12 per course.

Metamorphic Association (1977; originally Pre-natal Therapy
Association)
26 Chalcot Square, London NW1. Tel. 01-586 8269.
Aim: to treat, train and teach people in manipulation
and massage to relieve pre- and birth traumas causing
physical and psychological disturbances.

London and Counties Society of Physiologists (1919)
100 Waterloo Road, Blackpool FY4 1AW. Tel. 0253
403548.
Publishes directory of members: 900 (graduates of the
Northern Institute of Massage, plus other approved teaching bodies).

Northern Institute of Massage (1924)
100 Waterloo Road, Blackpool FY4 1AW. Tel. 0253 403548.
Courses: certificate in body massage and physical culture;
diploma in health and beauty therapy; diploma in remedial
(Swedish) massage – 4–12 months' home study, plus some
practical *or* about 4 months' attendance at the College.

Reflexology

Based on the principle that 'there is a direct reflex action between the nerve endings in the feet (and hands) and the various organs of the body'.

'Compton House'
87 High Street, Hampton, Middlesex. Tel. 01-979 3119.
Courses arranged on request (for 20 people).

Applied Kinesiology

Touch for Health (1976)
42 Worthington Road, Surbiton, Surrey. Tel. 01-399 7377.
Courses held in London and around the country in techniques of muscle testing to diagnose 'physiological conditions, and anatomical problems of the body', and methods of 'systematic balancing' of the body. Basic course (12 hours), seminars for 'professional therapists', lecture demonstrations.

Postural Integration and Pulsing

'Specialised forms of bodywork, using principles of connective tissue manipulation, Reichian and gestalt bodywork, acupuncture and movement awareness . . . to release the body from chronic and accumulated tension.'
Pulsing achieves 'release and integration of the mind, body and spirit' without physical pain. (Contact *The Open Centre* for details – see under 'Psychotherapy: Centres'.)

London Institute of Postural Integration (1978)
c/o 18 Park Hill Road, East Croydon, Surrey CR0 5NA. Tel. 01-680 4660.
Courses: 6-week basic training programme (200 hours).

6. ACUPUNCTURE

† British Medical Acupuncture Society (1980)
c/o 21 Aigburth Drive, Sefton Park, Liverpool L17 4JQ.
Tel. 051-728 7366.
Aim: 'to stimulate and promote the use and scientific understanding of acupuncture as part of the practice of medicine.' Members: 50.

The British College of Acupuncture (1964)
Registrar: 118 Foley Road, Claygate, Surrey. Tel. 78 64171.
Courses: 2-year part-time (16 weekends and practical) postgraduate, open mainly to doctors, dentists, physiotherapists, natural medicine practitioners, leading to LicAc. Students: 80; 3rd year for BAc. Students: 20.

British Acupuncture Association and Register (1960)
34 Alderney Street, London SW1V 4EV. Tel. 01-834 1012.
Publishes Register and Yearbook. Members: 368 (MBAcA), includes 174 overseas members mostly graduates of the British College of Acupuncture.

College of Traditional Chinese Acupuncture (1960)
Queensway, Royal Leamington Spa, Warwickshire CV32 5EZ. Tel. 0926 39347.
Courses: 2½-years full-time, leading to LicAc; further year for BAc. Students: 170.

Traditional Acupuncture Society (1977)
Queensway, Royal Leamington Spa, Warwickshire CV32 5EZ. Tel. 0926 22121.
Members: 80 MTAcS (students and graduates of the College of Traditional Chinese Acupuncture).

International College of Oriental Medicine (1971)
Green Hedges House, Green Hedges Avenue, East Grinstead RH19 1DZ. Tel. 0342 28567.
Courses: 3-year full-time leading to BAc. Students: 50;

some postgraduate courses (2 years) for DAc. Publishes an International Register of Oriental Medicine. UK practitioners: 10.

The Liu Academy of Taoist Therapies (1974)
13 Gunnersbury Avenue, Ealing Common, London W5. Tel. 01-993 2549.
Courses: 3-year part-time, includes foundation studies in t'ai chi, martial arts as well as traditional Chinese medicine (massage, herbal medicine, acupuncture, etc.). Students: 50.

7. RADIESTHESIA

† Psionic Medical Society (1968) and Institute of Psionic Medicine
Garden Cottage, Beacon Hill Park, Hindhead, Surrey. Tel. 042-873 5752.
Psionic medicine 'seeks to determine, by the use of the radiesthetic faculty, the cause of the imbalance and disharmony in the vital dynamic forces, resulting in disorder and disease' and the means of treatment. Journal. Members: 20 (qualified practising medical practitioners and dentists); 150 associates.

Delawarr Laboratories (1942)
Raleigh Park Road, Oxford. Tel. 0865 48572.
Radionic practice, treating 200 patients. Information service. Newsletter. Annual conference. Make and sell diagnostic and treatment instruments. Members: 800.

International College of Radionics (1947)
Highfield, Dane Hill, Haywards Heath, Sussex RH17 7EX. Tel. 0825790 214.
Correspondence courses (6 month – 2/3 years) in radionics, radiesthesia, dowsing, etc. Makes and sells radionic instruments, homeopathic remedy potentisers. Students: 1000 a year

Magneto-Geometric Applications
 3 The Hermitage, Westwood Park, Forest Hill, London
 SE23 3QD. Tel. 01-699 6604.
 Make and sell radiesthetic instruments e.g. homeopathic
 potency simulators, magneto-geometric radionic analyser,
 developed by the late Malcolm Rae.

The School of Radionics (1962)
 Brimfield Cottage, Brimfield, Ludlow, Shropshire SY8 4NE.
 Tel 058472 208.
 Courses: 18-month part-time, leading to MRadA. Students:
 37.

The Radionic Association (1943)
 16a North Bar, Banbury, Oxon OX16 0TF. Tel. 0295 3183.
 Aim: 'to protect and promote the practice of radionics as
 an honourable and skilled profession.' Keeps a register of
 practitioners. Lectures, conferences. Library. Journal. Members: 94 practitioners (qualifying from the School of
 Radionics); 460 associates.

8. HEALING

Orthodox Christian Organisations

Burrswood (1948)
 Groombridge, Nr Tunbridge Wells, Kent TN3 9PY. Tel.
 089276 353.
 Registered nursing home (30 beds), founded by the late
 Dorothy Kerin. Resident chaplain; services with laying on
 of hands; distant healing. International Fellowship – supports
 the work through prayer. Journal. Members: 2000.

The Christian Fellowship of Healing (1952)
 15 Chamberlain Road, Edinburgh EH3 7AL. Tel. 031-447
 9383.
 Aim: 'to restore healing to its rightful place in the normal
 ministry of the Church.' Distant healing, laying on of hands,

counselling. Members: 50 (non-denominational).

The Churches Council for Health and Healing (1946)
St Peter's Vestry, Eaton Square, Hobart Place, London
SW1W 0HH. Tel. 01-235 3305.
A committee representing the British churches and medical
and allied professions 'for mutual consultation and co-
operative action'. Member organisations: 24; guilds and
fellowships of healing in association: 10.

Divine Healing Mission (1908)
The Old Rectory, Crowhurst, Nr Battle, Sussex TN33
9AD. Tel. 042483 204.
Daily intercessions for healing; services with laying on of
hands. Residential accommodation for 30. Journal. Members: 450 (non-denominational); area representatives: 38.

Fountain Trust (1965)
3a High Street, Esher, Surrey KT10 9RP. Tel. 78 67331.
Charismatic renewal organisation. Information on world-
wide charismatic movement and its ministry of healing.
Meetings, conferences. Journal..

Guild of Health (1904)
Edward Wilson House, 26 Queen Anne Street, London W11
91B. Tel. 01-580 2492.
Aim: 'to restore the healing ministry of Christ through His
Church.' Intercession; counselling; lectures, conferences.
Journal. Members: 2000; local groups: 300 (UK and
abroad).

Guild of St Raphael (1915)
c/o All Saints Vicarage, 7 Margaret Street, London, W1N
8JG. Tel. 01-636 1788.
'Observe a rule of prayer, study and work' for the ministry
of healing. (Anglican). Journal. Members: 2000.

St Christopher's Hospice (1967)
   51 Lawrie Park Road, London, SE26. Tel. 01-778 9252.
   54 beds for the care of the dying. Research into the control
   of pain and other physical distress. *NB* there are 29 other
   such hospices in the country.

Other Healing Organisations

The following list is not meant to be exhaustive. It gives
examples of organisations concerned with distant healing,
hand healing, spiritualist healing, psychic healing.

The Atlanteans (1957)
   42 St George's Street, Cheltenham, Gloucestershire GL50
   4AF. Tel. 0242 25437.
   A New Age teaching network of 450 (UK and abroad).
   Healing groups; courses in healing; absent healing; hand
   healing. Journal. Members: 50.

The College of Psychic Studies (see under 'Centres')
   Distant healing groups. About 30 healers.

The College of Psycho-Therapeutics (1954)
   Stockland Green Road, Nr Tunbridge Wells TN3 8TT.
   Tel. 089286 3166.
   A centre for 'esoteric studies, colour research, spiritual
   therapies', founded by the late Ronald Beesley. 7-day
   courses in spiritual healing.

The Guild of Spiritualist Healers (1964)
   99 Bloomfield Road, Gloucester GL1 5BP. Tel. 0452 25455.
   A branch of the Spiritualist National Union. (Most of the
   healing takes place in Guild churches.) Annual conference.
   Members: 2100 – approved practising healers, trainee
   healers, SNU diploma holders (healing), associates.

The Harry Edwards Spiritual Healing Sanctuary Trust (1947)

Burrows Lea, Shere, Guildford, Surrey. Tel. 048641 2054. Absent and contact healing 'through attunement to . . . healing doctors in Spirit'. Journal (6000 subscribers).

The National Federation of Spiritual Healers (1955)
The Old Manor Farm Studio, Sunbury-on-Thames, Middlesex TW16 6RG. Tel. 76 83164.
Multi-denominational. Healer members may with permission give healing in 1500 NHS hospitals. Trains healers. Keeps directory of healer members. Newsletter. Members: 2000 healers; 600 probationers; 30 associates (doctors and paramedical practitioners).

The Seekers Trust (1925)
The Close, Addington Park, Nr Maidstone, Kent ME19 5BL. Tel. 0732 843589.
Community of about 30, holds prayer circles for healing every day (6000 names a week). Some guest flats for those wishing daily healing, or for retreat purposes. Journal. Members: 230.

The Spiritualist Association of Great Britain (1872)
33 Belgrave Square, London, SW1. Tel. 01-235 3351.
70 healers involved in running free clinic all week. Information on 23 Commonwealth Spiritualist Churches in UK, who have own healers.

Westbank Healing and Teaching Centre
(see under 'Centres')

The White Eagle Lodge (1936)
New Lands, Rake, Liss, Hampshire GN33 7HY. Tel. 073082 3300.
Spiritual healing according to White Eagle's guidance: laying on of hands, group prayer and thought-projection using colour ray healing; daily healing service. Teaches healing. 8 daughter Lodges. Journal. Members: 3000 (UK and abroad).

World Healing Crusade (1952)
  476 Lytham Road, Blackpool, Lancashire FY4 1JF. Tel.
  0253 43701.
  Worldwide network of prayer for the sick: Divine healing
  services, led by Brother Mandus around the UK and
  abroad; tapes on Divine healing, healing intercessions.
  Free magazine sent to 140,000.

9. PSYCHOTHERAPY-GROWTH (Eastern and Western approaches)

Psychotherapy

Association of Child Psychotherapists (1947)
  Burgh House, New End Square, London NW3. Tel. 01-450
  5014.
  The only professional association for child psychotherapists.
  Approves training given at 3 schools. Members: 200
  (accepted by the Training Council).

The following 5 organisations all train and certify practitioners:

British Association of Psychotherapists
  121 Hendon Lane, London N3 3 PR. Tel. 01-346 1747.

British Psycho-Analytical Society
  63 New Cavendish Street, London W1. Tel. 01-580 4952.

Institute of Group Analysis
  1 Bickenhall Mansions, Bickenhall Street, London W1. Tel.
  01-486 7657.

Society of Analytical Psychology
  30 Devonshire Place, London W1. Tel. 01-486 2321.

Association of Jungian Analysts
  19 Burgess Hill, London NW2. Tel. 01-435 7424.

Hypnotherapy

† British Society of Dental and Medical Hypnosis
10 Chillerton Road, London SW17. Tel. 01-672 3025.
Training courses: 3 weekends. Members: 1000.

Blythe Tutorial College of Hypnosis and Psychotherapy (1975)
Warwick House, Stanley Place, Chester. Tel. 0244 311414.
Part-time courses (held in Chester and London) in 4 units:
(i) hypnosis and applications (4 months); (ii) advanced
hypnosis and regression (6 months); (iii) psychodynamics (5
months); (iv) supervised work (6 months). Leads to membership of Association of Hypnotists and Psychotherapists.
Members: 40.

British Hypnotherapy Association (1958)
67 Upper Berkeley Street, London, W1. Tel. 01-723 4443.
Only admits graduates from the Psychotherapy Centre
(London). Courses: 4-year full-time.

British Society of Hypnotherapists (1959)
51 Queen Anne Street, London W1. Tel. 01-935 7075.
Practising members: 20 (MBSH). Courses discontinued.

Biofeedback, Relaxation, Autogenic Training

The Psycho-Biology Institute (1970)
c/o Audio Ltd, 26–28 Wendell Road, London W12. Tel.
01-743 1518.
Biofeedback, healing and holistic health. Courses: 10 weekly
seminars (10–12 students each).

Relaxation for Living (1972)
29 Burwood Park Road, Walton-on-Thames, Surrey. Tel.
98 27826.
Courses: 6 or 7 sessions, correspondence course available.
34 authorised teachers in the UK. Newsletter. Students:
500 a year.

Relaxation Seminars (1977)
   10 Pond Close, Hethersett, Norwich, Norfolk. Tel. 0603 811075. Course: 4 hours (Unit 1 of Silva Mind Control). 3 instructors in the UK (Sussex, Norfolk, Essex). Graduates: 300.

Centre for Autogenic Training (1978)
   12 Milford House, 7 Queen Anne Street, London W1M 9FD. Tel. 01-637 1586.
   Courses (on a group or individual basis): introductory (1 hour for 8 weeks 6–20 to a group), advanced work, according to individual needs.

Creativity Mobilisation Technique (1978) (address as above)
   Basic course: 6–8 weeks. Self development through 'no-form mess painting'.

Humanistic Psychology

Courses for Professional Training and Higher Education

Antioch Centre for British Studies (1973)
   115 Shepherdess Walk, London N1. Tel. 01-250 4011.
   Courses include individualised MA programme in humanistic psychology (18–39 months). Students: 64.

British Association for Bioenergetic Analysis (1978)
   Meeting House, University of Sussex, Falmer, East Sussex BN1 9QN. Tel. 0273 66755 ext. 296.
   Ongoing training programme for professionals in the caring professions. Also offer open weekend workshops, seminars, in counselling.

The Centre for Psychosynthesis and Education (1965)
   38 West Hill Court, Millfield Lane, London N6. Tel. 01-340 1612.
   An educational trust founded by the late R. Assagioli. Aim: to offer the principles and techniques of psychosynthesis (a transpersonal/spiritual psychology). Full public

programme and professional training programme (3 months–5 years). Students: 60 (full- and part-time).

Clinical Theology Association (1962)
Lingdale, Weston Avenue, Nottingham NB7 4BA. Tel. 0602 785475.
Courses: 1- and 2-year seminar courses in human relations, pastoral care and counselling held throughout the country (estimated 7000 have taken the 2-year course). Workshops in primal integration: a method of re-living birth in a 'clear dual consciousness'. Annual conference. Newsletter.

Institute of Biodynamic Psychology (1976)
Centre for Bioenergy, Acacia House, Centre Avenue, The Vale, Acton Park, London W3 7JX. Tel. 01-743 2437.
Short courses in biodynamic psychology; foundation course: 9 months; 3-year diploma course. A physiological approach to psychotherapy 'which makes for a biodynamic unification of the organism on psychic and somatic levels'. Journal. Students: 85.

Institute of Psychosynthesis (1973)
Highwood Park, Nan Clarks Lane, Mill Hill, London NW7. Tel. 01-959 3372.
Part-time courses for professional education. Counselling, information service. Journal. Students: 25.

The Institute for the Development of Human Potential (1978)
55 Tufnell Park Road, London N7. Tel. 01-607 9217.
2-year diploma courses in humanistic psychology – experience, theory and practice, held in London, Surrey and Nottingham. Occasional workshops. Students: 32 (London).

The Institute for Transactional Analysis (1974)
Upper Green, Hawkhurst-Sandhurst, Kent TN18 5JT. Tel. 058085 361.
Courses: introductory weekends (25 students); 4-day intermediate; 3–4-day advanced workshop; training days. Held in London and Northampton. Journal. Bulletin.

London Gestalt Centre (1974)
31 John Ratcliffe House, Chippenham Gardens, London NW6. Tel 01-328 9062.
Aim: to 'complete the client's experience and awareness of himself, in such a way that anxiety is reduced, emotional blocks removed, and the person's functioning and development can proceed more freely'. Courses: 7-week introductory programme; 1-year intensive training; 3-year training leading to qualification as a Gestalt Therapist.

Philadelphia Association (1965)
2 Eton Road, London NW3.
Training in psychotherapy and community therapy 3 years (min.). Students: 10. Study programme to 'examine the theory and practice of anthropology, meditation, phenomenology, psychoanalysis, yoga systems . . . seeking, perhaps through indirection to come to ourselves.' Students: 75 a term.

Polytechnic of Central London, Short Course Unit (1976)
309 Regent Street, London W1R 8AL. Tel. 01-580 2020 ext. 220.
Courses: dramatherapy, psychodrama, art therapy, dance, bio-energetics, creative groupwork, co-counselling. Students: up to 20 a course.

Westminster Pastoral Foundation (1969)
23 Kensington Square, London W8. Tel. 01-937 6956.
Courses: 1-year full-time (including counselling practice). Students: 25; 2-year part-time – students: 48; 1-year part-time (1 evening a week) for lay training in pastoral care and counselling – students: 40. Membership of Institute of Pastoral Education and Counselling – 3-year course.

Centres

Alive in Leeds (1979)
    8 Granby View, Leeds 6. Tel. 0532 780660.
    Evening classes, weekend and residential workshops in
    dance, gestalt, encounter, rebirthing, etc.

Beanstalk (1979)
    128 Byres Road, Glasgow G12 5HD. Tel. 041-339 2803.
    Workshops in Glasgow in postural integration and massage,
    natural dance, dramatherapy, gestalt, etc. Newsletter.

Centre for Transpersonal Psychology (1973)
    26a Gilston Road, London SW10 9FF.
    Workshops, counselling network and training programme
    for the 'development of human growth and potential and
    creative exploration of the psyche.'

The Growth Centre Tyneside (1977)
    54 St Georges Terrace, Jesmond. Newcastle-upon-Tyne.
    Tel. 0632 814860.
    Runs courses for professional training (communication
    skills, etc.), group work; offers counselling. Psychodrama,
    gestalt, transactional analysis courses.

Holwell Centre for Psychodrama (1975)
    Combe Cottage, Stonecombe, East Down, Barnstaple
    Devon. Tel. 027188 2209 (for bookings).
    Residential training courses in group therapy and psycho-
    drama; diploma course. 2–3 years part-time.

Humanistic Administrative Services (1978)
    21 Lyndhurst Road, London NW3. Tel. 01-435 6626.
    Facilities for gestalt, psychosynthesis, healing, acupuncture,
    biofeedback, rolfing, etc.

London Co-Counselling Community (1974)
    11 Brookside Gardens, Enfield, Middlesex. Tel. 01-976 0416.
    Courses: 40 hours basic training 'in simple techniques de-

signed to reach areas of stored up distress and to release it physically', and 'to develop a positive, celebratory attitude to oneself and to life'. Information also on Co-counselling International Network and Re-evaluation Counselling.

The Open Centre (1977)

188 Old Street, London EC1. Tel. 01-278 6783 (answering service).
Staff of 7 'committed to providing group and individual therapy at reasonable prices'. Classes in gestalt, bio-energetics, massage, dance, encounter, taido, postural integration, pulsing. Lectures.

The Pellin Centre (1976)

43 Killyon Road, London, SW8. Tel. 01-622 0148.
Weekend workshops, ongoing groups and individual counselling in contribution training and gestalt therapy.

Psychodrama and Sensitivity (Awareness) Training (1973)

83a Oxford Gardens, London W10. Tel. 01-969 7766.
Ongoing groups, weekend workshops, professional workshops and psychotherapy with individuals and couples; assertiveness training groups.

Whole Person Co-operative (1979)

85a Islip Street, London NW5. Tel. 01-267 8508.
A group of 9 trained by the late William Swartley and Jean Snow offering individual and group work in primal integration.

Sport

The Inner Game (1979)

204a West End Lane, London NW6 1SG. Tel. 01-794 9633.
Courses in Inner Tennis, and Skiing, Golf, etc. Aim: 'to help the player of life get in touch with the already self-existing process (of) . . . "natural learning".'

The Sporting Bodymind (1979)
Holcombe, Weald Way, Caterham, Surrey. Tel. 0883 42506.
Aim: 'to lead to better and more fulfilling sports performance.' Weekend workshops, individual consultancy,
residential courses, ongoing classes (London and Bristol)
using yoga, visual motor skill training, psychosynthesis, biofeedback.

Astrology

Astrological Association (1958)
36 Tweedy Road, Bromley, Kent. Tel. 01-464 3583.
International organisation. Conferences, meetings; journal
and newsletter – includes information on astrological groups
in the UK (15). Members: 450 (open).

British Astrological Psychic Society (1976)
49 Canham Road, South Norwood, London SE25. Tel.
01-771 3200.
Keeps list of 50 consultants (UK) in palmistry, tarot,
astrology. Newsletter. Members: 600 (open).

Faculty of Astrological Studies (1948)
37 Sherwood Court, Bryanston Place, London W1H 5FF.
Tel. 01-262 7548.
Correspondence course, leading to the certificate and
diploma examinations; evening classes; short courses.
Tutors: 16. Students: 450. Keeps list of qualified astrol-
ogers.

The Mayo School of Astrology (1973)
Piper's Wood, Leighton Drive, Beetham, Milnthorpe,
Cumbria LA7 7BE.
Correspondence courses: basic course (9–12 months); ad-
vanced course (leading to DMS Astrol.).

Centre for Transpersonal Astrology (1978)
Flat 5, 42 Belsize Park Gardens, London, NW3. Tel. 01-586
0059.

'A resource pool and a training workshop programme to help foster cross-fertilisation between . . . astrology and depth/transpersonal psychology.'

Yoga

Albion Yoga Movement (1972)
Flat 1a, 7 Rosecroft Avenue, London NW3. Tel. 01-435 3774. Integral yoga (also teach meditation, t'ai chi). Teacher training courses, lectures, seminars, retreats. 10 other yoga organisations affiliated.

B. K. S. Iyengar Teachers' Association
58 St Michael's Avenue, Bramhall, Stockport, Cheshire, SK7 2PG.
Keeps register. Members: 170.

British Wheel of Yoga (1965)
Glyn Galleries, Glyn Ceiriog, Llangollen, Clwyd. Tel. 0691 50912.
Teacher/instructor courses. Links with local education authorities. Information on groups, courses, organisations; publications. Emphasis on need for an integrated yoga, i.e. development on physical, emotional, mental and spiritual levels. Members: 3000.

The Yoga for Health Foundation (1978)
Ickwell Bury, Nr Northills, Biggleswade, Bedfordshire SG18 9EF. Tel. 076727 271.
Accommodation for 30 – can take the physically handicapped. Specialises in 'remedial, therapeutic and relaxation activities'; regular weekend and 5-day courses. Individual programmes also arranged. 40 regional clubs in UK.

Organisations for Meditation and Psychological/Spiritual Teachings

Eastern Traditions

Arica (1974)
    188 Old Street, London EC1.
    Training to bring about 'self-realisation and clarification
    of consciousness'. 3-day, 2-week and 40-day intensives.
    Members: 400.

Beshara (1971)
    Sherborne House, Sherborne, Nr Cheltenham, Gloucester-
    shire. Tel. 0451 448.
    8-month intensive courses in esoteric studies, meditation,
    contemplation, centred round the teachings of Ibnul 'Arabi
    (12th-century Islamic mystic). Students: 40 a year. 6
    regional centres.

British Meditation Society (1976)
    51 Aldridge Road, Villas, London W11. Tel. 01-229 8912.
    Aim: 'to enable ordinary people to combine deep spiritual
    realisations with an active and useful life'. Structured courses
    in meditation. Affiliated to the International Foundation for
    Spiritual Unfoldment. Members: 2500.

Buddhist Centres
    Apply: The Buddhist Society, 58 Eccleston Square, London
    SW1V 1PH. Tel. 01-828 1313.

The Gurdjieff Society (1950)
    11 Addison Crescent, London W14.
    Members: 700.

Kalptaru (1975)
    Top floor, 10a Belmont Street, London NW1. Tel. 01-485
    3216.
    Rajneesh meditation centre. 2-week introductory courses to
    Rajneesh's methods; courses in massage, meditation, re-
    flexology, bio-yoga, encounter, healing. 12 centres (UK).
    Members: 80,000 (world).

Raja Yoga Centre (1971)
    96–8 Tennyson Road, London NW6. Tel. 01-328 2478.
    Free courses of instruction in meditation; lectures, exhibitions. Part of the World Renewal Spiritual Trust: 11 centres (UK); 600 (world). Followers: 1,500 (UK).

The School of Meditation (1961)
    158 Holland Park Avenue, London W11 4UH. Tel. 01-603 6116.
    Training in meditation, using 'universal technique'. Centres in Sheffield, Basingstoke, Lincolnshire. Members: 600.

Sufi Orders

Chisti Order (founded by Hazrat Inayat Khan)
    Barton Farm, Bradford-on-Avon, Wiltshire.
    Aim: to become a centre for craft work, healing and natural medicine; to run courses and country-type festivals.

Idries Shah c/o Institute for Cultural Research
    PO Box 13, Tunbridge Wells, Kent. Tel. 089286 2045.

Theosophical Society in England (1875)
    50 Gloucester Place, London W1H 3HJ. Tel. 01-935 9261.
    Lectures and study groups on theosophical teachings 'the body of truths which forms the basis of all religions'. Branches in over 60 countries. Library, journals. Members: 2500.

Transcendental Meditation (1958)
    Roydon Hall, East Peckham, Nr Tonbridge, Kent CNT N12 5NH. Tel. 0622 813243.
    Courses: instruction in the TM programme (7 days), the Science of Creative Intelligence (30 lessons), TM Siddhi programme (12 lessons and 2 weeks residential for levitation and invisibility etc.); teacher training. International College; European Research University. Teachers: 400; centres: 80. Members: 106,000.

Western Traditions

For a comprehensive list and description of 135 retreat houses and places of monastic hospitality in the UK see *Away from it all*, Geoffrey Gerard, London 1978.

Information also available from: Association for Promoting Retreats, Church House, Newton Road, London W2. Tel. 01-727 7924.

Christian Science (1879)

106 Palace Gardens Terrace, London W8 4RT. Tel. 01-221 5650.

Founded 'to commemorate the word and works of our Master, which should reinstate primitive Christianity and its lost element of healing'. Churches and Societies in UK: 270; world: 3500.

Church of Scientology (1953)

St Hill Manor, East Grinstead, West Sussex. Tel. 0342 24571.

Centres in Manchester, Edinburgh, London, Plymouth. Courses: communications: students: 2000 a year; training in auditing (i.e., counselling) at various levels: students: 1000 a year.

EST Centre (1977)

81 Piccadilly, London W1. Tel. 01-491 2974.

Course: 2 weekend intensives (9–12 a.m. onwards) for about 250 people; postgraduate courses. Graduates: 1400.

Inner Light Consciousness in Europe

c/o The Moorhurst Centre, Holmwood, Dorking, Surrey RH5 4LJ. Tel. 0306 81033.

Workshops, lectures on 'Inner Light Consciousness'; evening and weekend intensives to 'develop the higher senses'; materials on Paul Solomon source readings (his teachings form the basis of the course). Newsletter. Graduates: 400.

Insight (1979)
   194a Sloane Street, London SW1X 9QX. Tel. 01-245 9788.
   Similar to but gentler than EST. Purpose to aid spiritual
   insight into oneself. Courses on demand.

Science of Mind Centre (1950)
   c/o Caxton Hall, London SW1. Tel. 01-352 4046.
   'A spiritual philosophy . . . based on the principle that there
   is but one infinite creative intelligence in all.' Instruction in
   practical techniques for applying to everyday life. Open
   lectures, courses; counselling, treatment.

Silva Mind Control (1972)
   131a St Julians Farm Road, Streatham Common, London
   SE27. Tel. 01-761 4765.
   Course: 4 units (10–12 hours each): (i) controlled relaxation; (ii) general self-improvement; (iii) effective sensory pro-
   jection; (iv) applied ESP. Graduates: 800.

10. ADDRESSES FOR AUSTRALIA, NEW ZEALAND, CANADA AND SOUTH AFRICA

General Organisations

AUSTRALIA:

Australian Natural Therapies Association
   729 Burwood Road, Hawthorn. Tel. 82 8714.

CANADA:

Consumer Health Organisation of Canada (1975)
   108 Willowdale Avenue, Ontario M2N 4X9. Tel. (416) 222
   6517.

SOUTH AFRICA:

'Consensus'
  PO Box 3150, Pretoria 0001. Tel. Pretoria 821323.
  Organises meetings for 64 New Age groups (health, healing, natural medicine).

Naturopathy

NEW ZEALAND:

New Zealand Association of Naturopaths and Osteopaths
  PO Box 26068, Auckland 3.

CANADA:

Ontario Naturopathic Association R.R.2
  Aurora, Ontario, Canada L4G 3G8.

Saskatchewan Association of Naturopathic Physicians
  Corner Board & 15th Regina, Saskatchewan.

SOUTH AFRICA:

High Rustenberg Hydro
  PO Box 2052, Stellenbosch, South Africa.

Herbal Medicine

CANADA:

Dominion Herbal College
  7527 Kingsway, Burnaby 3, British Columbia.
  Affiliated to the Canadian Herbalist Association of British Columbia.

Emerson College of Herbology
  815 Bancroft Street, Pointe Claire, Quebec, Canada H9R 4L6.

Appendix

Nutrition

New Zealand Vegetarian Society
  Box 454, Auckland.

CANADA:

Canadian Association for Preventive and Orthomolecular
Medicine
  2177 Park Crescent, Coquitlam, British Columbia, Canada
  V3J 6T1.

Canadian Health Food Association
  20440 Douglas Crescent, Langley, British Columbia, Canada
  V3A 4B4.

Music Therapy

NEW ZEALAND:

New Zealand Society for Music Therapy
  167 Wadestown Road, Wellington.

Natural Childbirth

CANADA:

International Childbirth Education Association
  182 Topcliffe Crescent, Fredericton, New Brunswick, Canada
  E3B 4P9.

SOUTH AFRICA:

Paramedical Association for Childbirth Education
  60 Valley Road, Parktown 2100, Johannesburg.

Homeopathy

AUSTRALIA:

Australian Institute of Homeopathy
7 Hampden Road, Artarmon 2064.

NEW ZEALAND:

New Zealand Homeopathic Society
Box 3929, Auckland 1.

CANADA:

Canadian Society of Homeopathy
Post Box 4333, Station 'E', Ottawa, Ontario K1S 5B3.
Tel. (613) 722 6603.

Osteopathy

AUSTRALIA:

Australian Osteopathic Association
71 Collins Street, Melbourne 3000.

Australian Chiropractors, Osteopaths and Natural Physicians
Association
6/102 Kirribilli Avenue, Kirribilli, NSW.

CANADA:

British Columbia Osteopathic Association
461 Martin Street, Penticton, BC.

Canadian Osteopathic Association
575 Waterloo Street, London, Ontario, Canada N6B 2R2.

Chiropractic

AUSTRALIA:

Australian Chiropractors Association
6 Pound Road, Hornsby, NSW.

NEW ZEALAND:

New Zealand Chiropractors Association
  PO Box 2858, Wellington.

CANADA:

Canadian Chiropractic Association
  1900 Batview Avenue, Toronto 17, Ontario.

SOUTH AFRICA:

The Chiropractic Association of South Africa
  29 Union Club Buildings, 69 Joubert Street, Johannesburg.

Acupuncture

AUSTRALIA:

Acupuncture Association of Victoria
  126 Union Road, Surrey Hills, Victoria 3127.

Acupuncture College of Melbourne
  296 High Street, Preston, Melbourne.

Psychotherapy-growth

NEW ZEALAND:

Psychotherapists and Hypnotherapists Institute of New Zealand
  1st Floor, Hampton Court, Wellesley Street, Auckland 1.

Association of Teachers of Transcendental Meditation
  192 Willis Street, Wellington.

Theosophy in New Zealand
  10 Belvedere Street, Epsom, Auckland 3.

Yoga Institute of New Zealand
  Box 904, Auckland.

CANADA:

Canadian Academy of Psychotronics
  43 Eglinton Avenue East, Suite 803, Toronto, Canada
  M4P 1A2.

Cold Mountain Institute
  Granville Island, Vancouver, BC V6H 3M5.
  (Encounter, acupuncture, gestalt, art therapy, etc.; BA MA
  courses.)

Canadian Institute of Psychosynthesis
  3496 Marlowe Avenue, Montreal, Quebec, Canada H4A
  3L7.

School of Hatha Yoga
  1984 Yonge Street, Toronto 7, Ontario.

Sufi Order
  9631 106a Avenue, Edmonton, Alberta T5H 0T2.

York University
  The Centre for Continuing Education and Growth Opportunities
  4700 Keele Street, Downsview, Ontario, Canada M3J 2R0
  (courses and workshops in biofeedback, bioenergetics,
  hypnosis, transactional analysis, yoga, etc.).

AUSTRALIA:

Raja Yoga Centres
  NSW: 531a Willoughby Road, Willoughby 2068; *Victoria*:
  33 Brunswick Street, Fitzroy, 3065 Melbourne.

Australian Biofeedback Society
  PO Box 7030, Sydney, 2001 Australia.

Sivananda School of Yoga
    3rd Floor, Embassy Place, 240 Bree Street, Johannesburg.

11. FURTHER SOURCES OF INFORMATION

Festival for Mind-Body-Spirit (1977)
    159 George Street, London W1. Tel. 01-723 7256.
    Aim: 'to encourage a greater networking of information
    about New Age activities and to encourage the greater
    participation of local organisations.' Organises regional
    festivals. Keeps a list of stall holders.

Human Potential Resources (1978)
    35a Station Road, Hendon, London NW4. Tel. 01-202 4941.
    Quarterly handbook containing a compendium of different
    natural therapy approaches. Mailing list: 5000.

Index

Index

Index

Fontana Paperbacks

Fontana is a leading paperback publisher of fiction and non-fiction, with authors ranging from Alistair MacLean, Agatha Christie and Desmond Bagley to Solzhenitsyn and Pasternak, from Gerald Durrell and Joy Adamson to the famous Modern Masters series.

In addition to a wide-ranging collection of internationally popular writers of fiction, Fontana also has an outstanding reputation for history, natural history, military history, psychology, psychiatry, politics, economics, religion and the social sciences.

All Fontana books are available at your bookshop or newsagent; or can be ordered direct. Just fill in the form and list the titles you want.
